How to
Survive
Dental
Performance
Difficulties

T0176983

How to Survive Dental Performance Difficulties

Janine Brooks MBE
DMedEth, MSc, FFGDP(UK), MCDH,
DDPHRCS, BDS, FAcadMEd

WILEY Blackwell

This edition first published 2018
© 2018 John Wiley & Sons Ltd

All rights reserved. No part of this publication may be reproduced, stored in a retrieval system, or transmitted, in any form or by any means, electronic, mechanical, photocopying, recording or otherwise, except as permitted by law. Advice on how to obtain permission to reuse material from this title is available at http://www.wiley.com/go/permissions.

The right of Janine Brooks to be identified as the author of this work has been asserted in accordance with law.

Registered Offices
John Wiley & Sons, Inc., 111 River Street, Hoboken, NJ 07030, USA
John Wiley & Sons Ltd, The Atrium, Southern Gate, Chichester, West Sussex, PO19 8SQ, UK

Editorial Office
9600 Garsington Road, Oxford, OX4 2DQ, UK

For details of our global editorial offices, customer services, and more information about Wiley products visit us at www.wiley.com.

Wiley also publishes its books in a variety of electronic formats and by print-on-demand. Some content that appears in standard print versions of this book may not be available in other formats.

Limit of Liability/Disclaimer of Warranty
The contents of this work are intended to further general scientific research, understanding, and discussion only and are not intended and should not be relied upon as recommending or promoting scientific method, diagnosis, or treatment by physicians for any particular patient. In view of ongoing research, equipment modifications, changes in governmental regulations, and the constant flow of information relating to the use of medicines, equipment, and devices, the reader is urged to review and evaluate the information provided in the package insert or instructions for each medicine, equipment, or device for, among other things, any changes in the instructions or indication of usage and for added warnings and precautions.While the publisher and authors have used their best efforts in preparing this work, they make no representations or warranties with respect to the accuracy or completeness of the contents of this work and specifically disclaim all warranties, including without limitation any implied warranties of merchantability or fitness for a particular purpose. No warranty may be created or extended by sales representatives, written sales materials or promotional statements for this work. The fact that an organization, website, or product is referred to in this work as a citation and/or potential source of further information does not mean that the publisher and authors endorse the information or services the organization, website, or product may provide or recommendations it may make. This work is sold with the understanding that the publisher is not engaged in rendering professional services. The advice and strategies contained herein may not be suitable for your situation. You should consult with a specialist where appropriate. Further, readers should be aware that websites listed in this work may have changed or disappeared between when this work was written and when it is read. Neither the publisher nor authors shall be liable for any loss of profit or any other commercial damages, including but not limited to special, incidental, consequential, or other damages.

Library of Congress Cataloging-in-Publication Data

Names: Brooks, Janine, author.
Title: How to survive dental performance difficulties / Janine Brooks.
Description: Hoboken, NJ : Wiley, [2018] | Includes bibliographical references and index. |
Identifiers: LCCN 2018010419 (print) | LCCN 2018010645 (ebook) | ISBN 9781119255635 (pdf) |
    ISBN 9781119255628 (epub) | ISBN 9781119255611 (pbk.)
Subjects: | MESH: Dentistry–standards | Professionalism | Work Performance–standards
Classification: LCC RK56 (ebook) | LCC RK56 (print) | NLM WU 21 | DDC 617.6–dc23
LC record available at https://lccn.loc.gov/2018010419

Cover Design: Wiley
Cover Image: ©yewkeo/Getty Images

Set in 9.5/12pt Minion by SPi Global, Pondicherry, India

Printed in Singapore by C.O.S. Printers Pte Ltd

10 9 8 7 6 5 4 3 2 1

Contents

viii **Contents**

Foreword

Becoming a member of the dental professions involves considerable personal effort, intellectual challenge, financial cost and emotional engagement. It is a great achievement and just the start of a privileged and rewarding career. Individuals are expected to consistently deliver what they have learned, to the best of their ability, for the benefit of patients, whilst adopting a persona and lifestyle that comply with ever higher public expectations and changing clinical practice and regulatory requirements, until they retire perhaps 40 years later.

Of course, none of us is perfect. We are human. Life happens. Things go wrong. We make mistakes. We all sometimes get tired, suffer physical or mental illness, have relationship or money problems. We are distracted by personal issues or family pressures, get bored or complacent or disillusioned by the system we work in, or are irritated by some of the people we work with or treat. Consequently, we take our eye off the ball. We may find we can't do some of the technical aspects of dentistry as well as we should or used to, or fail to earn as much money as we expected, while doing what the public and profession expect of us. Patients now complain more frequently than before and their expectations are increasingly high, fed both by our own profession's sophisticated marketing and glossy advertisements and better public information about what standards to reasonably expect.

How we deal with all this *stuff* is important to our survival. It's tempting to ignore any niggling self-doubts and only concentrate on the aspects of dentistry we are comfortable with, or to blame others when things go awry. We need, however, to acquire and maintain not only the confidence and skills to manage the great juggling act of great dentistry, but also the humility to acknowledge our weaknesses, seek and listen to proper advice and ask for the right sort of help.

A letter of complaint from a patient, threat of legal action from a solicitor or a notice from the GDC or other regulator telling us we are under investigation can either be the start of a personal catastrophe or an opportunity to review how we manage work and life and get back on track.

Dr Janine Brooks, who is herself a dentist, has unique knowledge and experience of supporting colleagues who have struggled or come under the spotlight and scrutiny of professional regulators over many years. This excellent book is a comprehensive guide to performance in dentistry that should be considered as a guide to prevention as well as cure and is essential reading for all dental professionals.

Helen Falcon MBE

Acknowledgements

I have been incredibly fortunate to have received contributions from several dental professionals who have generously written their fitness to practise stories in the spirit of altruism and a desire to help other dental professionals. I am very grateful to them all and I believe their words bring home the humane aspects of what it is to struggle with performance.

I am also extremely grateful to a non-dental professional who has contributed so generously of his time, John Brooks, my husband. He has tirelessly proof read the manuscript and offered a much-needed sanity check, allowing me to see the wood for the trees, not to say practise (verb) for practice (noun). Any inadvertent errors are mine alone.

Acknowledgements

Abbreviations

BDA	British Dental Association
BDDG	British Doctors and Dentists Group
COPDEND	Committee of Postgraduate Dental Deans and Directors
COSHH	Control of Substances Hazardous to Health
CPD	Continuing Professional Development
CQC	Care Quality Commission
DDU	Dental Defence Union
DHSP	Dentists' Health Support Programme
DHST	Dentists' Health Support Trust
DPL	Dental Protection Ltd
DRO	Dental Reference Officer
DRS	Dental Reference Service
GDC	General Dental Council
GMC	General Medical Council
GPC	General Pharmaceutical Council
HEE	Health Education England
HIW	Healthcare Inspectorate Wales
HSCB	Health and Social Care Board
HSE	Health and Safety Executive
IOC	Interim Orders Committee
LDC	Local Dental Committee
LETB	Local Education and Training Board
MBTI	Myers–Briggs Type Indicator
MDDUS	Medical and Dental Defence Union of Scotland
MHRA	Medicines and Healthcare Products Regulatory Agency
NCAS	National Clinical Assessment Service
NES	NHS Education for Scotland
NHSE	NHS England
NIMDTA	Northern Ireland Medical and Dental Training Agency
NLP	Neuro-Linguistic Programming
ORE	Overseas Registration Examination

PAG	Performance Advisory Group
PCC	Professional Conduct Committee
PCSE	Primary Care Support England
PDP	Personal Development Plan
PHP	Practitioner Health Programme
PLDP	Performers Lists Decision Panel
PPC	Professional Performance Committee
PSA	Professional Standards Authority
PSD	Practitioner Services Division
RDSPB	Regulation of Dental Services Programme Board
RIDDOR	Reporting of Injuries, Diseases and Dangerous Occurrences Regulations 2013
RQIA	Regulation and Quality Improvement Authority
TKI	Thomas–Kilmann Conflict Mode Instrument
TRaMS	Training, Revision and Mentoring Support Programme
VBR	Values-based recruitment

Chapter 1 **The basics of performance**

Introduction

This book has been written to help those dental professionals who have struggled with their performance, are struggling, might struggle or are supporting colleagues who are struggling. That is probably just about the whole dental profession at some point in a working career. It will be of use to all categories of dental professional, clinical and non-clinical.

For a number of years, I have worked with dental professionals who have been referred to the General Dental Council (GDC). This has largely been in the capacity of providing advice, coaching or mentoring support to individuals. Over my career, I have worked with and supported dental professionals who have been deemed poor performers. I was instrumental in setting up the National Clinical Assessment Service (NCAS) systems for dentistry and I worked as an Associate Postgraduate Dental Dean supporting dentists in difficulty. I regularly coach or mentor dentists who are facing GDC hearings or local performance procedures. I have also been responsible for developing and implementing training and managing teams of dentists who supported colleagues undertaking programmes of remediation. Before all that, I was a Clinical Director of Community Dental Services for almost 20 years and directly responsible for a large staff and occasionally I had to deal with staff who performed poorly. I'm not the most experienced in these areas, but I consider myself to have a very good knowledge and experience over 30+ years.

All this experience has led me to want to write this book that I hope will help others who come into contact with remediation in whatever guise. Primarily, it provides information that would be helpful should you personally find yourself the subject of a GDC investigation. It will also be of help to those who support professionals under investigation, whether that be with regulation or with an organisation, and here I have called on my experience of developing training programmes for coaches/mentors, educational supervisors, trainers and appraisers. It is my hope that it may also be of interest to dental

How to Survive Dental Performance Difficulties, First Edition. Janine Brooks.
© 2018 John Wiley & Sons Ltd. Published 2018 by John Wiley & Sons Ltd.

professionals involved in fitness to practise panels. Here, the analysis of how processes affect those individuals referred and the case studies of colleagues may assist in humanising our regulation.

Finally, all dental professionals should find the book of use in the spirit of prevention. It is a sobering thought that any dental professional could be the subject of a GDC referral and investigation at any stage of their career – none of us is immune. During their long careers, dental professionals will interact with many, many patients, and making errors is far more common than is admitted. If you are a dental professional working in a non-clinical field, you can still be referred to the regulator, so you cannot assume that fitness to practise does not apply to you.

I have worked with issues of performance for a number of years both nationally and locally. My input has been strategic in setting up systems and processes, but also operational in that I have personally worked with many dental professionals who find themselves struggling and with a complaint against them, and I still do. My response to performance has always been that any dental professional could find themselves in this position and that few actively seek to perform badly or unprofessionally. Dentistry is a complex profession and the vast majority of dental professionals try every day to do the best work they can for the benefit of others and in the best interests of their patients. Things can go wrong for a wide variety of reasons but in my experience, a proactive, humanistic approach is much more likely to lead to resolution than a punitive reaction. Some dental professionals can find themselves more at risk of struggling and I have included a section on taking a preventive approach in Chapter 7, which includes case studies.

The book will cover reasons why dental professionals get into difficulties; issues of professionalism and underpinning culture and ethics; the regulatory processes and mechanisms within which UK dental professionals work, including the General Dental Council, the Care Quality Commission (CQC) and equivalents in Scotland, Wales and Northern Ireland, and commissioning arrangements. Also included will be information about organisations who work with individuals who struggle; the processes of the GDC when investigating and hearing a complaint; the tools that professionals can use to help them to improve performance; and how self-awareness and insight can be deepened. In addition, I have included some case studies of dental professionals who have first-hand experience of struggling and being involved in fitness to practise processes. Many, if not all of the tools, instruments and mechanisms I have included will be of use to all dental professionals in the course of their day-to-day dental practice. The final chapter considers the skills that supporters of colleagues who struggle need to develop as well as some useful one-to-one techniques.

I firmly believe that the vast majority of dental registrants have no desire to perform at less than their best. I also believe that every one of us has performed poorly during our working careers. We have all had bad days, bad weeks possibly even bad years when our performance has slipped. I'm not suggesting that all dental professionals put patient safety at serious risk but we have all produced work that could be judged as less than the best. We have all exhibited behaviour that we regretted when viewed in hindsight. The reasons for this are many and varied and I will cover those in Chapter 2. In this respect, poorly performing dental professionals are an issue for every one of us; we could all become poor performers and it is something in which we all have a part to play. We all need to be vigilant for colleagues who struggle, not to castigate them, not to point the finger and breathe a sigh of relief that it's them and not us, but to support and help them. We are a caring profession and we should extend that care to each other. If we don't care for our colleagues, how can we really care for our patients? It is not possible to have a dual approach without demonstrating a degree of hypocrisy.

What is performance?

Before I take a closer look at performance concerns, dips or difficulties, it seems appropriate to first consider what performance is. A good place to begin might be to look at definitions of performance.

> **Performance**:   'The execution or fulfilment (of a duty, etc.)'
> 'The act or process of performing or carrying out'
> **To perform**:   'Carry into effect, be the agent of'
> (Oxford English Reference Dictionary, 1996)

If performance and performing are about carrying out an act, then for dental professionals that act must be dentistry, in all its forms. The duty that requires execution or fulfilment must be providing dental services for others, most usually patients. So let's take a look at definitions of dentistry:

> **Dentistry**:   'The profession or practice of a dentist'

It seems to me that this definition is not very helpful.

> **Dentist:**   'A person who is qualified to treat the disease and conditions that affect the mouth, jaws, teeth and their supporting tissues'
> (Oxford English Reference Dictionary, 1996)

Whilst this may be a definition of the most recognisable aspect of dentistry, it fails to cover the richness of roles that dental professionals undertake in the broader field of services to patients, the public and society.

Does that bring us any closer to what dental performance is? Probably a little, but it doesn't get to the essence or spirit of what performance actually is, let alone what satisfactory performance, competent performance, acceptable performance, good performance, excellent performance, underperformance or poor performance is. Every act, intervention or conversation undertaken by a dental professional, in the operation of their role, is performed. Each can be judged to be either acceptable or unacceptable. Performance is the essence of dentistry.

The nine principles of *Standards for the Dental Team* (GDC, 2013) set out what dental registrants must do to maintain their registration with the General Dental Council. They are the standards against which all dental professionals are judged. They can be deemed to be our standards of performance. On page 3 of *Standards for the Dental Team*, performance is explicitly noted.

'This document sets out the standards of conduct, performance and ethics that govern you as a dental professional. It specifies the principles, standards and guidance which apply to all members of the dental team. It also sets out what patients can expect from their dental professionals.'

The *Business Dictionary* (2017) defines performance as:

'The accomplishment of a given task measured against preset known standards of accuracy, completeness, cost, and speed'.

It seems to me that this is getting closer to defining performance for dental professionals. I'm going to take the definition apart a little further.

Task: The performance of an aspect of dentistry, be that clinical or non-clinical. For this example, I will use a new patient examination (Table 1.1).

I think we are getting closer to what performance includes. However, the example above shows largely human factors relating to a specific individual. Performance is wider than the single individual undertaking a task; other factors or variables affect the ability of an individual to perform any given task at any given time. The personal characteristics of the dental professional will affect their ability to undertake tasks. I will cover character in Chapter 3. In the case of a clinician, this ability is

Table 1.1 Mapping a new patient examination to the *Business Dictionary* definition.

Criteria	Preset known standard
Accuracy	FGDP (UK) Clinical Examination
Completeness	Examination of hard tissues, soft tissues (intra- and extraoral)
	Full history to include dental, medical, personal and sociobehavioural
	Reason for attendance/attitude to dental health
	Special investigations
Cost	Unit of Dental Activity (UDA) value. NHS Band 1 (as at 16 August 2017) £20.60
Speed	10–15 minutes

compounded by factors relating to the individual patient. I will go into more detail about external factors in Chapter 2. In addition to the personal characteristics of the professional and patient, there are other external factors, for example the environment and context in which work is undertaken.

Another point to remember is that the performance of any one professional can never be wholly good or wholly poor. If everything dental professionals do is a performance, then some things will be undertaken to a higher level or a poorer level of performance than others. It is interesting to ponder which aspects of performance are more likely to be interpreted by our patients as poor.

In their dental advice series *Handling Complaints England*, Dental Protection Ltd (2016) states:

> 'Communication skills, and in particular non-verbal skills, significantly affect a patient's satisfaction level towards outcomes of treatment. Providing patients with extra time during treatment changes their perception of the level of care provided. Research shows that patients are more likely to sue if they feel rushed and that insufficient time has been spent with them.'

It is not really surprising that patients are more likely to judge their care on the non-clinical aspects of the dentistry they experience. However, dental professionals can often underestimate how important these aspects are to patients. Patients expect their dental professionals to be clinically competent, of course. They do not expect to be treated without respect, courtesy or to feel unduly rushed.

In their research into public attitudes to dental standards, Costley and Fawcett (2010) found that:

'The most significant issue relating to standards that arose from these discussions was that of communication. Communication is important in its own right. Moreover, it appears to underpin every other issue and concern arising in the discussions and its importance cannot be overemphasised in the standards review.'

Communication is a subject that includes an array of subtle factors. Poor communication features in many of the cases heard by GDC fitness to practise panels. Chapter 3 will consider communications in greater detail.

Having briefly considered what performance is, I will now turn to think about poor performance.

What is poor performance?

As I have noted previously, performance is what we do every day as dental professionals. You perform whether you are clinical or non-clinical, general dental practitioner or dental public health consultant, full-time researcher or indemnity adviser. It's what professionals do – they perform. I do not use the terminology in any way to suggest a lack of integrity or reduced authenticity.

If performance is what dental professionals do, what is poor performance? A little simplistic maybe, but it is performing at less than the acceptable standard as expected by our commissioners and professional regulators, the CQCand the GDC. Ethically and morally, I think poor performance can also be considered as working below what is expected in providing a safe, acceptable standard of care for patients. If you no longer work clinically with patients then the standard is what is expected of the role you occupy or by your employer or commissioner. However, there is more to the GDC nine principles than clinical care and all registrants must meet the principles.

The National Clinical Assessment Service (2010) has a helpful definition of poor performance.

'Any aspects of a practitioner's performance or conduct which:
- *pose a threat or potential threat to patient safety;*
- *expose services to financial or other substantial risk;*
- *undermines the reputation or efficiency of services in some significant way;*
- *are outside acceptable practice guidelines and standards.*

Any performance concern has the potential to impact on patient safety or impinge on the wider public interest so the particular circumstances and risks associated with each case must be systematically evaluated. Performance concerns may relate to a single area of concern or be multi-factorial. Areas of concern include clinical errors, knowledge or skill deficits, outdated forms of practice, inappropriate attitudes/behaviour or conduct, dishonesty and other unlawful activity, poor interpersonal communication, as well as health and addiction problems.'

This is a useful definition of poor performance. It shows that the term encompasses a breadth of issues and also hints at the complexity of poor performance. The range is considerable; in my experience, concerns are rarely simple even if they appear so when they first come to notice.

How does poor performance develop? If we knew the answer to that question with certainty, then prevention would be so much more straightforward. Sadly, reliable crystal balls are hard to come by. However, I think the quote below goes some way towards an explanation.

> *'The things we have done in the past become our future.'* (Te Ao Pehi
> Kara, Maori spiritual expert, Tokanaga)

I came across this quotation when visiting the Wellington Museum on a trip to New Zealand and it resonated strongly with me. It seems to me that often poor performance is the result of a slow accumulation of 'just below par' ways of working, each building on the last until eventually the performance exhibited by an individual is poor and unacceptable. It is a slow descent down a slippery slope almost imperceptible on a day-to-day basis. As the quotation suggests, what we did yesterday and today will become our future. Of course, there are also the one-off events that occur. These can often be serious. Interestingly, I think that the one-off serious issue can be dealt with more quickly and successfully than the slow descent. Possibly the reason is that one-off issues are more visible than the slide.

The document *Handling Concerns about the Performance of Healthcare Professionals* (NCAS, 2006) included a list of concerns that define poor performance.

- Low standard of work; for example, frequent mistakes, not following a task through, inability to cope with instructions.
- An inability to handle a reasonable volume of work to a required standard.
- Unacceptable attitudes to patients.
- Unacceptable attitudes to work or colleagues, for example, unco-operative behaviour.
- Poor communication, inability to acknowledge the contribution of others.

- Poor teamwork, lack of commitment and drive.
- Poor punctuality and unexplained absences.
- Lack of skills in tasks/methods of work required.
- Lack of awareness of required standards.
- Consistently failing to achieve agreed objectives.
- Acting outside limits of competence.
- Poor supervision of the work of others when this is a requirement of the post.
- A health problem.

If this is a list of concerns, then perhaps the reverse will shed light on what satisfactory or good performance includes, for example a good awareness of required standards, only acting within limits of competence and handling a reasonable volume of work to a required standard. The list may also illuminate which aspects of performance are more likely to be unacceptable to patients. These will probably include those non-clinical skills such as unacceptable attitudes to patients and poor communication raised by Costley and Fawcett (2010).

> 'There are three rules you should live by. Be on time. Learn your lines.
> Don't be a dick. It boils down to respecting people's integrity and choices,
> being professional and accepting you are not the centre of the universe.'
> (Interview with Fionn Whitehead, actor, 2016)

I really liked this quote when I read it; it seemed to me that it has resonance for all dental professionals. In fact, I liked it so much that I mapped it into the nine GDC professional standards (Table 1.2), just to help me think it through.

Perhaps if the GDC adopted the rules from Fionn's quote, dental professionals would find it easier to remember the basic tenets of the service we provide. This may seem rather a 'tongue in cheek' comment, but I hope it will be taken in the spirit I intend, using humour to make a serious point.

Every dental professional will experience difficulties, every dental professional will make mistakes. It's not the difficulty or the mistake that really matters, it's what the individual does next that proves their mettle. Those who are humble in knowing themselves, recognise when their performance dips and do something about it will move forward stronger. Those who are arrogant and ignore their mistakes or don't even appreciate they have made mistakes are much more likely to experience a regulatory investigation. Unfortunately, this is not as simple as it might at first appear. Later, in Chapter 8, I will be considering the work of Kruger and Dunning (1999) and their findings in the field of insight.

Table 1.2 Mapping the GDC professional standards to Fionn Whitehead quote.

Quote rules	Fionn's interpretation	GDC standard
Be on time	Respecting people's integrity and choices	Put patients' interests first Obtain valid consent Maintain and protect patients' information
Learn your lines	Being professional	Communicate effectively with patients Maintain, develop and work within your professional knowledge and skills Raise concerns if patients are at risk
Don't be a dick	Accepting you are not the centre of the universe	Have a clear and effective complaints procedure Work with colleagues in a way that is in patients' best interests Make sure your personal behaviour maintains patients' confidence in you and the dental profession

Fitness to practise

Here I will briefly add some preliminary thoughts about fitness to practise, which is covered in more detail in Chapters 4 and 6.

Fitness to practise is an overarching concept which includes a number of aspects. A dental professional who is fit to practise is able to provide dental services, care and treatment safely and effectively to others in society. This includes the professional's ability to undertake procedures and interventions – that is, their clinical ability and competence, skill, knowledge and expertise. It also includes behaviour and character traits demonstrated in both the practising environment and outside.

Sometimes when you become involved with performance or fitness to practise processes, it can seem easier to ignore the issues and tell yourself they will go away on their own. This can be a reaction that is hard to resist but it is a strategy that rarely if ever works. It is the same whether you are the registrant about whom there has been a complaint or if you become involved in proceedings. I have worked with a number of registrants who have ignored letters from the GDC and done nothing, sometimes even to the point of a hearing being conducted in their absence. Once an issue has been flagged, it will progress, regardless of whether the registrant engages with the process or not. Refusal to co-operate and engage with the fitness to practise mechanisms does little to predispose the GDC panel toward your case. It can be difficult, but doing nothing and turning away will not work.

Red door/green door

Referral to the GDC generally follows one of three pathways.
1. No substance, no case to answer.
2. Some or all of the complaint has substance. The professional accepts that, recognises the wake-up call and uses the process to improve their practice, emerging from the situation bruised but a better professional.
3. Some or all of the complaint has substance. The professional refuses to recognise or appreciate this and rails against the complaint and the GDC. This approach can result in a very poor outcome for the professional.

The GDC lays considerable store on registrants demonstrating 'insight'. Where insight is absent or poorly demonstrated, it shows that the individual is unable to detect that a problem has occurred. Their self-awareness is so low that they believe their practice or attitude or behaviour is acceptable and change is unnecessary. Occasionally, self-awareness and insight are at such a low level that the individual may actually think their performance is good and everyone is against them. In cases where insight is minimal or absent, the GDC cannot feel assured that the issues or failures will not be repeated. Hence the outcome is likely to be harsher, sometimes severe.

Those registrants who follow route 3 can face the Red Door, which opens onto the world outside dentistry. Step through the Red Door and you are no longer able to call yourself a dental professional. You have been erased from the Dental Register. All that training and education gone for ever. Your lifestyle changed for ever. You are an ex-dental professional. It seems unbelievable that this should be a choice for any dental professional and yet, so many contribute to their own passage through the Red Door. Is this arrogance, stupidity, a certain belief in their own rightness? It's difficult to tell. Occasionally, I use a coaching technique where the coach takes the coachee to a future place, in this case to think about a life outside dentistry. What would that look like? How would it feel? What would your lifestyle be? Would your relationship with your spouse and children change? Sometimes, this technique can be the jolt needed and reality is glimpsed. I believe that insight and self-awareness are so important I have devoted Chapter 8 to the subject.

Errors occur in healthcare literally all the time. Dentistry is no different. We dental professionals all make mistakes regularly. If you don't think you do then my response to you is 'Yes you do, although you may not have sufficient insight to realise you do'. If you make a mistake, realise you have made a mistake and learn from it, then you are on the road to being a successful practitioner. I'm not excusing mistakes, particularly those that directly harm patients; mistakes cost money and money is scarce. Most mistakes or errors are underpinned by a multitude of factors, perhaps the most significant being the human, the dental professional.

The Dental Defence Union (2015) reported a 110% increase in clinical negligence claims between 2011 and August 2015, with rises of 10% each year. Patient expectations may be a factor in this increase. Ensuring that patients are fully aware of what their treatment entails can help to encourage realistic patient expectations. This is part of good communication and it underpins informed consent. Discussions with patients should always include risks, outcomes and consequences. This is particularly important in the case of cosmetic interventions.

When thinking about the performance of dental professionals, it can be interesting to consider the expressed level of satisfaction which patients report. The King's Fund (2017) published data showing that the level of public satisfaction with NHS dentistry is up to 61%. This is an increase of 7% since 2015 and the highest level of satisfaction since the early 1990s. The underpinning data are taken from the British Social Attitudes Survey

References

Business Dictionary (2017) Definition of performance. Available at: www. businessdictionary.com/definition/performance.html (accessed 8 January 2018).

Costley, N. and Fawcett, J. (2010) *Public and Patient Attitudes*. George Street Research, Edinburgh.

Dental Defence Union (2015) *Increase in Clinical Negligence Claims*. www.theddu.com/press-centre/press-releases/dento-legal-climate-worsening-says-ddu (accessed 9 January 2018).

Dental Protection Ltd (2016) *Dental Advice Series – Handling Complaints, England*. www.dentalprotection.org (accessed 8 January 2018).

General Dental Council (GDC) (2013) *Standards for the Dental Team*. General Dental Council, London.

King's Fund (2017) *Public Satisfaction in the NHS and Social Care in 2016. Results and Trends from the British Social Attitudes Survey*. Available at: www.kingsfund.org.uk/publications/public-satisfaction-nhs-2016 (accessed 8 January 2018).

Kruger, J. and Dunning, D. (1999) Unskilled and unaware of it: how difficulties in recognizing one's own incompetence lead to inflated self-assessments. *Journal of Personality and Social Psychology*, 77, 1121–1134.

National Clinical Assessment Service (NCAS) (2006) *Handling Concerns about the Performance of Healthcare Professionals – Principles of Good Practice*. Available at: www.ncas.nhs.uk/publications

National Clinical Assessment Service (NCAS) (2010) *Handling Performance Concerns in Primary Care*. Available at: www.ncas.nhs.uk/publications
Oxford English Reference Dictionary (1996) Oxford University Press, Oxford.
Whitehead, F. (2016) Interview. *Big Issue*, **October 24–30**, p. 35.

Further Reading

General Dental Council (GDC) (2014) Annual Report. Available at: www. gdc-uk.org
General Dental Council (GDC) (2015) Annual Report. Available at: www. gdc-uk.org

Chapter 2 Background and contributory factors: how performance issues can arise

Introduction

In Chapter 1, I stated that almost every dental registrant, no matter which professional group they belong to, will have performed at less than their best at some point in their career. Dental professionals are only human and humans make mistakes, professionals have bad days and are certainly not perfect. However, society expects more from its professionals than the rest of the population and we have to accept that and be forever watchful of our own performance.

However, clinical performance is not the only aspect of our fitness to practise that we must constantly consider; behaviour is also critical for professionals. Again, society expects its professionals to demonstrate an enhanced standard or level of behaviour; what society may tolerate when displayed by a non-professional will not be tolerated when displayed by a professional. These behaviours and attitudes can be encapsulated in the term 'professionalism'.

In this chapter, I will look at the background to poor performance and factors that contribute to individuals' failure to undertake their role to an acceptable standard. I highlight processes that are in place to deal with poor performance, the support that is available and ways in which poor performance can be minimised. I think it's also important to understand that it is probably impossible to eradicate poor performance in human beings. It may be that we should not attempt to eradicate poor performance as that is how we learn. Learning from experience and particularly when things do not go to plan is the essence of reflective practice and the reflective practitioner. If we were all perfect, what would there be to learn? Chapter 10 includes a section on reflection, reflective writing and reflective models.

Perhaps we need to understand performance better, encourage professionals to develop their self-awareness and insight, undertake true reflective practice and concentrate on deliberate acts of negligence and harm.

How to Survive Dental Performance Difficulties, First Edition. Janine Brooks.
© 2018 John Wiley & Sons Ltd. Published 2018 by John Wiley & Sons Ltd.

A little history might be of interest to illuminate contributory factors to performance and how they have evolved over the years. In 1955, the last year of the Dental Board of the United Kingdom and just before the formation of the GDC, 13 fitness to practise cases were considered by the Board, with three registrants erased; two of those cases were initially heard in 1954 (Dental Board of the United Kingdom, 1957). In 1956, dental regulation came out from under the wing of the General Medical Council (GMC) and stood alone as a regulatory body – the General Dental Council. At that time, there were 15 895 dentists registered with the GDC. Other dental professional groups were not regulated by the Dental Board of the UK when it separated from the GMC. Dentistry was different in those days and the way fitness to practise was handled was also different. Perhaps as important is that society was different and the attitude of the public to the dental profession was different, as patients may have been less likely to make a complaint against their dentist.

In 1955, the 13 cases heard by the disciplinary committee covered the following areas of professional misconduct.

1. False certification; wrongfully obtaining money from NHS authorities; failure to supply dentures
2. Obtaining credit by fraud
3. Canvassing; failing to provide treatment; wrongfully claiming and receiving money (erased)
4. Gross indecency with male persons
5. Negligence as director of body corporate
6. Indirectly advertising or canvassing
7. Driving motor car while under influence of drink; dangerous driving
8. Advertising
9. Canvassing
10. Wrongfully claiming money from employer
11. Covering *
12. Wrongfully receiving money under NHS Acts; driving motor car while under influence of drink or drugs
13. Covering *
* There is no definition or explanation for this term.

Two of the 13 cases concerned clinical issues and both of those cases involved non-clinical issues in addition.

In 2016, there were 41 483 dentists registered and in that year, a total of 308 fitness to practise cases (of dentists) were heard. Chapter 6 covers fitness to practise cases in more detail.

Pressures on dentists

Working in dentistry can be stressful and pressured (Figure 2.1). Many factors can contribute to a dental professional performing at less than their

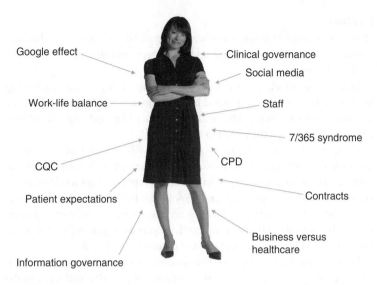

Google effect

Clinical governance

Social media

Work-life balance

Staff

7/365 syndrome

CQC

CPD

Patient expectations

Contracts

Business versus healthcare

Information governance

Figure 2.1 Pressures on dental professionals.

best. Some professionals cope better than others and coping will be affected by life factors. If the individual is healthy and happy with a good home life then they are likely to be more able to withstand pressures and stresses than someone who is unwell, unhappy and with a chaotic home life.

Factors that underpin poor performance

Poor performance is a complex and complicated issue and the factors that underpin it reflect this. Patel *et al.* (2011) published a summary of a recent literature review in which they provide a comprehensive picture of the factors influencing poor performance in dental practitioners. It is rare to find a single cause, and this makes analysis of the problem and subsequent remediation a real challenge. However, it is important to find out what has contributed to the poor performance exhibited by an individual because if the causes are unknown, rectifying the problem becomes much more difficult. If analysis of the contributory factors is either not undertaken or done badly then the chances of a successful remediation are diminished. This would be akin to beginning to treat a patient without a thorough examination and diagnostic tests. It sounds obvious and yet all too often a thorough review of underpinning issues and contributory factors is not applied when trying to uncover why a dental professional is struggling. A reason for this may be the emphasis laid on 'human' factors, an example of which would be clinical skill or lack of it displayed by a clinician. In this chapter I'll look at some of the factors that underpin poor performance, both intrinsic and extrinsic, in more detail.

Health

Ill health in dental professionals is well reported, with numerous studies into physical and mental health and addiction problems that can beset those working in dentistry.

Dentists are notoriously a 'hard to reach' group when it comes to accessing healthcare because they can often be reluctant to seek treatment for their personal health problems. Thus it is imperative to find out more about how best to assist them on their road to recovery.

Kemp and Edwards (2015) report on a 2013 British Dental Association survey of work-related stress in UK dentists. The results indicated that 39% of community dentists and almost half of GDPs reported high levels of stress, compared to an average of around 15% for all British workers. Of course, self-reported levels of stress alone do not automatically indicate ill health. People deal with stress in many ways with varying coping strategies. However, levels of reported stress can indicate the potential for ill health.

In 2014, the BDA carried out two further studies looking into the stress and well-being of member dentists, comparing the results with levels in the UK general adult population. One study included community dentists, the second dentists working in general practice.

First, let's look at the survey of dentists working in community dental services to identify levels of stress and well-being and assess the current state of those services. It was administered online to 1643 community dentists who were members of the BDA. Of these, 554 responded, yielding a response rate of 34%. Of these, 481 were confirmed to be working as community dentists. The key findings from the two studies were that for both sectors, almost half the dentists who responded to the survey reported low levels of life satisfaction and a similar proportion reported low levels of happiness. For both sectors, community and general practice, there was a strong relationship between perception of health and work-related stress. Dentists who reported high levels of stress at work were significantly less likely to report that they were in good health. The surveys also compared dentists with the general population and found that the reported level of well-being in dentists was much lower than the general adult UK population. The study concluded that:

'... *exposure to high levels of stress at work is likely to be an important factor driving dentists' overall levels of personal well-being ... The occupation-specific pressures that dentists experience may help to explain why they report lower levels of life satisfaction and higher levels of anxiety compared with adults in the UK population.*'

According to current evidence, health professionals, and in particular dentists, have a higher than average risk compared to the general population of suffering from mental health problems (Brooks *et al.*, 2013; Rada and Johnson-Leong, 2004), suicide (Alexander, 2001; Meltzer *et al.*, 2008; Sancho and Ruiz, 2010) and substance misuse problems (Curtis, 2011; Kenna and Lewis, 2008; Kenna and Wood, 2005).

There is extensive evidence to suggest that poor mental health can have detrimental effects on a person's overall physical health, social health and quality of life (BDA, 2015; MacDonald *et al.*, 2005), hence the significance of maintaining good overall mental health. From an employment perspective, being mentally well underpins the ability to work.

Not only is dentistry considered a highly stressful career (Myers and Myers, 2004) but it is also perceived as more stressful compared to other occupations (Moore and Brodsgaard, 2001). Dentists are academic high achievers as evidenced by the grades needed to gain a place in dental school. They can often be perfectionist in character, which is good for undertaking detailed, technical procedures. However, this character trait can trigger mental health problems such as depression (Accordino *et al.*, 2000), particularly if problems arise at work, and dentists can often be in denial of this (Stoddard Dare and DeRigne, 2010).

Given that dentists, through their training and practice, attain a degree of health knowledge, it would be expected that this would enhance their overall health. However, studies suggest the opposite; dentists, along with other health professionals, not only possess the knowledge of how to harm themselves, they can also access a means of doing so (Coombs, 1996). In order to be held in high regard, some dentists hide their addictions and mental health problems, often because of lack of insight or perception; they are afraid that they will be disciplined or dismissed from their position.

Clinical knowledge and expertise
Whilst lack of clinical knowledge and skills is perhaps the most easily recognisable factor underpinning poor performance, it is also often the factor that responds most readily to remediation. Dentistry is an extremely technical profession and new ways of doing things, new technologies, new kit, new materials bombard us almost daily. It is very difficult to keep up and practitioners can often become out of date without realising it. Falling behind with changes, new developments and new ways of working can happen within a very few years of qualifying, probably less than might be thought.

Isolation can compound compromised clinical knowledge and expertise. If professionals do not meet up with colleagues and talk about the latest 'thing' then they can deceive themselves that they are still on top of their game. Whilst reading journals and completing online continuing professional development can help, these are rarely sufficient. Dentists need to talk to other dentists, sharing new ideas and techniques. Face-to-face training and education enable participants to learn not only from the tutor or presenter but also from other participants. The degree of actual knowledge transfer in a face-to-face situation is far higher than having information pushed via an online source.

When reviewing fitness to practise cases and determinations, it is interesting to see that many of the cases involving clinical knowledge and expertise include basic clinical dentistry. A high proportion of cases show deficiencies in examination and treatment planning, caries diagnosis, radiography, periodontal examination and treatment. These are not new techniques. Could it be that dental professionals seeking CPD ignore the basics because they believe they know them? Perhaps it is more exciting to attend courses on new techniques or those that may enhance the business rather than 'wasting' time on repeating old knowledge. However, even 'old knowledge' changes. Record keeping is a very good example of changes over the years. I shudder to think what my records were like 30+ years ago. Another example is ensuring patient engagement to underpin good communication and consent. The rise of bioethics and the weight placed by society on individual autonomy make the ability to engage patients in their own care and work in partnership an essential skill. Basics do change and what was once acceptable practice is no longer; if a dental professional fails to keep up to date with basic, routine dentistry, they place their patients and themselves at risk.

Environment/context

Of all the factors that underpin performance, environment and contextual factors may be the least well understood. The impact on the individual is particularly poorly understood.

These are external factors that may or may not be under the direct control of the dental professional. If the environment, the dental surgery, clinic, hospital or educational establishment a person works in is poor or even toxic, it is unlikely that he or she will flourish and produce work of a satisfactory standard, let alone good work. The environment in which we work can be a contributory factor to less than acceptable performance and, importantly, a good environment can be the tipping point for turning poor performance around.

Those who struggle and are working in a good, supportive, nurturing environment are often quickly helped to turn around any problems and get back on track. Conversely, those who struggle and work in a poor or even toxic environment generally receive no help, or indeed the wrong 'help', and can spiral down into repeated poor performance with little prospect of finding the right track.

Factors that are part of the work environment include the following.

- Teamwork; a well-functioning team that works together effectively and efficiently can do much to reduce stress on individuals.
- Professional isolation, including networking and support mechanisms.
- Workload, including quantity and ability to control one's own workload.
- Financial issues.
- Working with challenging patients.

Behavioural/attitudinal factors

Of all the underpinning factors that can contribute to poor performance, perhaps the most powerful is the behaviour of the professional. It is also the most difficult to change or remediate. Behaviour is underpinned by the character traits of the individual and develops at an early stage in our life, often before school.

Harrison-Evans and Krasodomski-Jones (2017) suggest that individual character traits, such as empathy, self-control, compassion, honesty and civic participation, seem generally to affect specific types of behaviour or reasoning. Broadly speaking, individuals scoring highly on each of these character traits were less likely to engage in negative behaviours, and more likely to take others into consideration when thinking about what course of action to take.

Learning for Life, a major research project largely funded by the John Templeton Foundation and Porticus UK (Arthur, 2009), focuses on the age range 3–25 years, which makes the scope and approach unique. The overall sample involves tracking more than 4000 children and young people, 300 parents and 100 teachers over a 2-year period in Birmingham, Bristol, Canterbury and London, together with a series of group interviews and case study observations. Two of the key findings were as follows.

- It was generally agreed that good character implied good morals and right behaviour.
- The primary influence on values was stated to be family, most particularly the mother, although the father was not infrequently mentioned. Travel and meeting different types of people made a significant impact.

The research is compelling that character traits are largely fixed by the time we begin our working life. However, whilst character and personality are major factors underpinning behaviour, they are not the only one. Impacts on the behaviour of an individual can be seen from both internal and external sources.

Figure 2.2 shows factors that can affect an individual and their behaviour, either positively or negatively. The magnitude of a factor, factors combining together or acting simultaneously will affect the actual behaviour manifested. An important aspect to consider when working with a colleague who may be

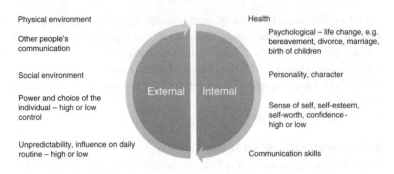

Physical environment

Other people's communication

Social environment

Power and choice of the individual – high or low control

Unpredictability, influence on daily routine – high or low

External　Internal

Health

Psychological – life change, e.g. bereavement, divorce, marriage, birth of children

Personality, character

Sense of self, self-esteem, self-worth, confidence - high or low

Communication skills

Figure 2.2 Factors that affect behaviour.

struggling with behavioural issues is what incentives or rewards they might be experiencing by exhibiting the behaviour. For some, there can be considerable rewards for acting 'badly' that they may not wish to relinquish. In such cases, the key is to either find an incentive to behave 'better' that gives a greater payback or to demonstrate that the current behaviour, if continued, will result in something of greater value being lost, for example registration.

This section defines a flavour of just how complex and complicated understanding the behaviour of an individual can be. However, with determination and a willingness to change on the part of the individual, it is possible to correct behavioural problems, even the most serious aspects. I expand further on character and virtue in Chapter 3.

Patient factors

Most dental professionals work with members of society – their patients. Each patient will bring their own unique set of characteristics, foibles, needs, demands and requirements. Patients are a cross-section of society; some are easy to get along with, others have difficulty accepting dental care. A few patients can be very challenging, either because of the complex dental care they require or because of the behaviours and attitudes they present in the dental practice. A very few patients can be demanding in a way that can adversely affect the dental team, and the professional–patient relationship. I have worked with dentists who have undertaken treatment at the insistent request of the patient that in hindsight was not the best thing to do.

Patients are now much more knowledgeable about what types of dental care are available. This knowledge comes from many sources: friends and family, online sources, magazines and television programmes. The adage that 'a little learning is a dangerous thing' can ring very true in some cases. Patients are not dental professionals who have spent years learning and honing practical skills, and patients rarely understand the underlying reasons why certain treatments may not be the right choice for them. Patients are often very busy people who may wish their treatment to be undertaken quickly, not being willing to make several appointments. For some dental professionals, it can be difficult to maintain the degree of assertiveness required not to succumb to the demands of patients. It is almost always wrong to try to meet misplaced patient expectations, as these instances are often when complications arise and treatments fail. The patient will forget the pressure they brought to bear on the dental professional to undertake the treatment requested in the timeframe set. It will be the professional who has to deal with a complaint.

Patients can be demanding, sometimes unreasonably or unrealistically. They can request treatments that are not appropriate and expect timescales that are not achievable. A registrant who allows themselves to be unduly influenced to undertake a treatment that they know to be detrimental to the oral health of their patient has started down the slippery slope of poor performance. In a similar way, the registrant who allows their patient to dictate treatment timeframes places themselves at serious risk of disappointing the patient and a disappointed patient is far more likely to make a complaint, possibly to the GDC.

Culture

Culture can be thought of as a system of fundamental values and beliefs set up by the 'founders'. By founders, I mean the people who established an organisation or practice or department. Culture is implicit and difficult to get to grips with. It's about shared assumptions about how things are done and can be summed up as: 'What we do around here'.

The culture of an organisation/practice is widespread; within a dental practice, the culture would be felt by all staff, no matter how large the practice. Dental corporate bodies and other large dental organisations will have their own culture that will have been determined by those who originally set them up.

Culture is extremely difficult to alter and will withstand changes in management and even ownership. New people become 'infected' by the culture and continue to nurture it. If the culture is supportive and chimes with those of individuals working in the organisation then it will exert a positive impact on the ability of professionals to perform well. If the culture is not supportive or is at odds with the values and beliefs of the professionals, then it will exert a negative impact on people working in the organisation and their ability to perform well.

Another aspect of culture to consider is that if everyone in a practice operates in a particular way, it can be very hard to push back and work differently. After trying to make changes that are met with resistance or even hostility, many professionals stop trying to alter things and just adopt the practice ways of working. Doing the right thing when everyone around does not takes a very strong person.

While the Francis Inquiry (2013) does not attribute the entire problem in Mid Staffordshire to the character of the trust's staff, its comments raise interesting questions concerning the relationship between the character of individuals, the culture of organisations and the quality of service that organisations provide.

Climate

The climate of an organisation or practice is all about the behaviour and attitudes of those who work there. It's 'how it feels around here'.

You can walk into a practice and immediately sense whether happy people work there or the reverse if no-one is talking to each other. Climate, unlike culture, doesn't have to be organisation or practice wide because it's all about the individuals. Groups of people within a practice can generate their own climate and the climate of a group is heavily influenced by who is a member of the group. Unlike culture, it is much easier to change climate. A large organisation may demonstrate a number of climates.

Work–life balance

This term is used frequently to indicate the proportion of our lives that we spend on different aspects of our existence. I've always found it a strange term as for me, work is part of my life, not outside it. I prefer to think of just balance. Do I have the correct split (for me) on what I think of as work, what I think of as home, family, friends, hobbies, etc.? This will vary on a regular basis. The important thing is that it's right for me and I keep checking that it is. Invariably, I find I spend less time visiting my mother than I would like to. There are friends I haven't seen for a very long time, but I still regard them as friends and try to keep in contact. I love the many aspects of my work, they give me tremendous satisfaction and I spend a considerable amount of time on work activities. Because I enjoy them so much and derive so much satisfaction from them, work isn't a chore; sometimes it's hard to think of what I do as work.

Balance will not be the same for everyone; in fact, it would be surprising if it were. We each have to explore what makes up the whole of our life and whether we spend the right amount of time on specific aspects. If we need to make room for something new, perhaps a postgraduate degree, then we will need to cut down on other aspects for a while. Those with children or grandchildren will want to ensure that the amount of time they spend with their children is right for them, the children and other family members.

The message is, make space to reflect on how you spend your time. Is it right? If not, how can you rebalance what you do to get closer to your ideal? Be realistic – we can't spend all our time on leisure activities if there is no money coming in. We can't expect a happy home life if we spend all our time at work or the gym or on the golf course. Working with a coach to help you uncover what you want from your life and how you want to be is time well spent. You can then focus on achieving the balance that is right for you.

I read a fascinating piece by Cokelet (2016) on work–life balance and whether this was an ethical luxury or a necessity. It got me thinking about how his suggestions might apply to dentistry and dental professionals. The premise was that lack of balance can contribute to corrosion of character. This struck a chord for me in the work I do providing coaching and mentoring for dental professionals in remediation. Several of the dentists I work with and have worked with described a lack of balance between work and non-work parts of their life. A number worked exceptionally long hours, taking on unreasonable contractual arrangements and stretching themselves to breaking point. Some were experiencing serious home life and family challenges and distractors. For several, there was a definite corrosion of character. What do I mean by this? Things like diminishing integrity, acting dishonestly and losing sight of putting patients' interests first.

Character traits are generally considered to be formed early on in our lives, possibly even before school. They are also generally considered to be fixed; that is, they do not change and, most importantly, when looked at in the context of remediation, they cannot be changed. There is a school of thought within healthcare regulation that to act dishonestly is a fundamental character flaw that cannot be remediated. However, if we accept that external factors can lead to a lack of balance and this can underpin a corrosion of character and lead to us acting 'out of character', then perhaps there is hope for remediation. Perhaps if we can remove those things that are causing the corrosion then we can rebalance. Character traits may well be formed early in our lives, but the experiences we have during our lives are constantly changing and surely these must have an effect on the translation of our character into behaviour. The key factor is whether the effect, the corrosion, is permanent or whether we can reverse the process.

Emotional state

An area that is often ignored as a contributory factor in poor performance is the emotional state of the registrant. For example, when there are problems at home, perhaps with partners, children or frail parents, this can distract us at work. Our emotional state can affect our ability to reason, the mind can wander or concentration dips. Such lapses are risky when providing patient care. When we are emotionally low, it can affect our ability to resist inappropriate demands from patients or staff.

The way we feel at home can affect work and the way we feel at work can affect home. The effects can be either positive and affect us in a good way, increasing our emotional resilience, or affect us in a negative way, sapping our emotional resilience. Being stressed at home can undermine our ability to work to the standard we wish to achieve. We are not robots who are always able to keep home and work in separate compartments. Dentistry is a stressful occupation and it takes superhuman strength to remain detached from that stress. I would go as far as to say it is impossible to be unaffected over the long years of a career. Whilst clinical dentistry has obvious stressors linked to patient care, staff management, financial management and business balance, other branches of dentistry can be equally stressful. Regardless of the work dimension, all dental professionals will have non-work stresses and challenges to their emotional resilience.

When we are emotionally in a low state and our resilience is reduced then we can find it harder to cope with stressors and external pressures. Strengthening and building emotional resilience is important in being able to cope with vulnerability and what life throws at us. There are a considerable number of factors that can be a source of stress and pressure. Any of these can make the difference between coping and not coping.

Maslach *et al.* (1996) developed an inventory underpinning three key aspects of burnout: emotional exhaustion, depersonalisation (a cynical detached feeling towards patients) and a reduced sense of personal achievement.

Chipchase *et al.* (2017) built on Maslach's work on burnout and concluded that:

> 'Dentists' anxiety in clinical situations does affect the way that dentists work clinically, as assessed using the newly designed and validated Dentists' Anxieties in Clinical Situation Scale (DACSS). This anxiety is associated with measures of burnout and decision-making style.'

They also reported that there were no studies looking at the effects of anxiety, stress or burnout on clinical decision making or clinical errors in dentists.

Maslach *et al.* (1996) suggested that the three key aspects of burnout can be found singly, but they also interact and that emotional exhaustion can lead to depersonalisation and together these two aspects contribute to a reduced sense of personal achievement. In my personal experience of mentoring and coaching dentists who have been referred to the GDC, emotional exhaustion plays a role, sometimes a significant role, in their susceptibility to dips in performance.

References

Accordino, D.B., Accordino, M.P. and Slaney, R.B. (2000) An investigation of perfectionism, mental health, achievement, and achievement motivation in adolescents. *Psychology in the Schools*, **37**, 535–545.

Alexander, R.E. (2001) Stress-related suicide by dentists and other health care workers. Fact or folklore? *Journal of the American Dental Association*, **132**, 786–794.

Arthur, J. (2009) *Graduates of Character. Values and Character: Higher Education and Graduate Employment*. Jubilee Centre, University of Birmingham.

British Dental Association (BDA) (2014) *Sources of Stress among Community Dentists*. BDA Research Findings No. 4. British Dental Association, Cardiff.

British Dental Association (BDA) (2015) *Dentists' Perceptions of Their Own General Health*. British Dental Association, Cardiff.

Brooks, S.K., Gerada, C. and Chalder, T. (2013) Doctors and dentists with mental ill health and addictions: outcomes of treatment from the Practitioner Health Programme. *Journal of Mental Health*, **22**(3), 237–245.

Chipchase, S.Y., Chapman, H.R. and Bretherton, R. (2017) A study to explore if dentists' anxiety affects their clinical decision-making. *British Dental Journal*, **222**(4), 277–290.

Cokelet, B. (2016) Work–life balance: luxury or ethical necessity? *Psychology Today*. Available at: www.psychologytoday.com/blog/questions-character/201606/work-life-balance-luxury-or-ethical-necessity (accessed 9 January 2018).

Coombs, R.H. (1996) Addicted health professionals. *Journal of Substance Misuse*, **1**, 187–194.

Curtis, E.K. (2011) When dentists do drugs: a prescription for prevention. *Today's FDA*. Available at: www.dentistwellbeing.com/pdf/DentistsDoDrugs.pdf (accessed 9 January 2018).

Dental Board of the United Kingdom (1957) *Minutes with Reports of Committees, etc. for the Year 1956 and General Index to the Minutes 1921–1956*. Vol. **XV**.

Francis, R. (2013) *Report of the Mid Staffordshire NHS Foundation Trust Public Inquiry. Executive Summary*. Stationery Office, London.

Harrison-Evans, P. and Krasodomski-Jones, A. (2017) *The Moral Web: Youth, Character, Ethics and Behaviour*. Demos. Available at: www.demos.co.uk/wp-content/uploads/2017/09/DEMJ5689-The-moral-Web-ethics-and-behaviour-on-social-media-170908-WEB-3.pdf (accessed 9 January 2018).

Kemp, M. and Edwards, H. (2015) *Psychosocial Working Conditions and Work Related Stress among Community Dentists in the UK*. British Dental Association, London, pp. 17–19.

Kenna, G.A. and Lewis, D.C. (2008) Risk factors for alcohol and other drug use by healthcare professionals. *Substance Abuse Treatment, Prevention and Policy*, **3**, 3.

Kenna, G.A. and Wood, M.D. (2005) The prevalence of alcohol, cigarette and illicit drug use and problems among dentists. *Journal of the American Dental Association*, **136**, 1023–1032; erratum 1224.

MacDonald, R., Shildrick, T., Webster, C. *et al.* (2005) Growing up in poor neighbourhoods: the significance of class and place in the extended transitions of 'socially excluded' young adults. *Sociology*, **39**(5), 873–891. Available at: http://dx.doi.org/10.1177/0038038505058370 (accessed 9 January 2018).

26 How to survive dental performance difficulties

Maslach, C., Jackson, S.E. and Leiter, M.P. (1996) *Maslach Burnout Inventory*, 3rd edn. Consulting Psychologists Press, Palo Alto, CA.

Meltzer, H., Griffiths, C., Brock, A., Rooney, C. and Jenkins, R. (2008) Patterns of suicide by occupation in England and Wales: 2001–2005. *British Journal of Psychiatry*, **193**, 73–76.

Moore, R. and Brodsgaard, I. (2001) Dentists' perceived stress and its relation to perceptions about the anxious patients. *Community Dentistry and Oral Epidemiology*, **29**, 73–80.

Myers, H.L. and Myers, L.B. (2004) 'It's difficult being a dentist': stress and health in the general dental practitioner. *British Dental Journal*, **197**, 89–93.

NHS Employers (2014) *Stress in the Workplace*. Available at: www.nhsemployers.org/ your-workforce/retain-and-improve/staff-experience/health-work-and-wellbeing/ protecting-staff-and-preventing-ill-health/taking-a-targeted-approach/emotional-wellbeing/stress-in-the-workplace (accessed 9 January 2018).

Patel, R., Eaton, E.A., Garcia, A. *et al.* (2011) Factors influencing dental practitioner performance: a summary of a recent literature review. *Oral Health and Dental Management*, **10**(3), 119–130.

Rada, R.E. and Johnson-Leong, C. (2004) Stress, burnout, anxiety and depression among dentists. *Journal of the American Dental Association*, **135**, 788–794.

Sancho, F.M. and Ruiz, C.N. (2010) Risk of suicide amongst dentists: myth or reality? *International Dental Journal*, **60**, 411–418.

Stoddard Dare, P.A. and DeRigne, L. (2010) Denial in alcohol and other drug use disorders: a critique of theory. *Social Work Faculty Publications*, **19**. http:// engagedscholarship.csuohio.edu/clsowo_facpub/19

Further Reading

Arthur, J., Kristjansson, K., Thomas, H. *et al.* (2015) *Virtuous Medical Practice*. Research Report. Jubilee Centre, University of Birmingham.

National Clinical Assessment Service (NCAS) (2011) *Factors Influencing Dental Practitioner Performance: A Literature Review*. Available at: www.ncas.nhs.uk/ publications.

Chapter 3 **Professionalism**

'We must remember that intelligence is not enough. Intelligence
plus character – that is the goal of true education.'

(Martin Luther King Jr, 1948)

What is professionalism?

Professionalism is an interesting word describing an interesting concept. In
this chapter, I will explore the concept in more depth. Those who are registered with the GDC are dental professionals and are required to act with
professionalism. But it's not easy to define what professionalism really is:
what it encompasses, how professionals should behave in an ever-changing
society, society's expectations of professionals and the character traits that a
professional should display. I will address some of these issues and questions
in this chapter. In addition, I will include some thoughts on the cultural and
ethical framework in which professionals operate in the UK.

There are certain characteristics that are said to characterise a profession
(Cook *et al.*, 2013).

- Provides a valued and valuable public service.
- Requires members of the profession to have knowledge and skills acquired
  by lengthy training.
- Has an ethical code of conduct.
- Requires autonomous thought in complex situations.
- Self-regulating.

These characteristics are relatively easy to demonstrate for the profession of
dentistry, with the possible exception of self-regulation, which has taken
rather a knock in the past few years. In 1956, when the GDC was first formed
as a stand-alone regulator, the issues of training for dentists and an appropriate ethical code of conduct were noted in the Chairman's address. The establishment of the GDC contributes one aspect of autonomy for the profession.
At its birth, any dentist could stand for election to the committee provided

How to Survive Dental Performance Difficulties, First Edition. Janine Brooks.
© 2018 John Wiley & Sons Ltd. Published 2018 by John Wiley & Sons Ltd.

that no fewer than 12 dentists nominated them. A number of additional seats were appointed by various bodies. The process is different today.

The professional who demonstrates autonomous thought in complex situation:

- carries out appropriate actions
- acts within boundaries
- is trusted
- uses 'practical wisdom', that is, knowledge acquired over the years.

Again, it is not hard to apply these characteristics to dental professionals. However, when considering performance, some have failed in their demonstration of those characteristics.

Looking at the characteristics of what constitutes a profession, given above, then what is professionalism? It's a word that encapsulates a great deal; for example, it will include:

- standards of conduct
- rules
- virtues.

Standards of conduct for the dental professional can be found in the nine principles set out by the GDC (2013). Rules include legal requirements as well as guidelines and frameworks constructed by regulators and specialist professional societies. Virtues are intrinsic qualities, traits and characteristics of the individual.

All societies have norms of behaviour that everyone in that society is expected to comply with, often called communal norms, for example not to steal. In addition, special groups in society have specific morality, also known as role morality. Role morality can be applied to healthcare professionals. It encompasses behaviour not usually shared by the general population and holds the profession to a higher standard than the rest of the community. Role morality includes:

- values and virtues that the rest of the populace feels that professional group should demonstrate, for example confidentiality
- that they are ambassadors or role models within the community.

Role morality applies to the person's whole life. It is not possible to segregate professional and private life. If a person is undisciplined in their private life, it will affect how they are perceived in their professional (public) life.

Being a professional means taking on very specific moral responsibilities. Professionals are obligated by the same moral standards as everyone else in society, the communal norms, but in addition, the professional function makes a number of strict demands on behaviour and character. Professionals are bound by both the uniqueness (for example, patients' interests first) and strictness (for example, honesty) of a higher moral standard than non-professionals.

Unique obligations are those not normally encountered by others. Dental professionals take on both unique obligations and stricter obligations and we agree to them by assuming the role. If a professional neglects their children, writes a bad cheque or cheats on their taxes, there is a moral and legal objection. The grounds of those objections are standards applied to everyone and there is not a sense that the professional has let society down specifically in regard to their specific role. Or is there? The functional line between professional and private is not a 'hard' boundary. Do beliefs about a professional's moral conduct outside the professional context have effects on their ability to be a professional? There is an argument that the conduct of dental professionals outside their work environment does affect the image of the profession; this could be called reputation. Society expects its professionals to be moral, ethical individuals who operate at that level in all dimensions of their life.

Certainly, our professional regulator believes that our conduct outside the sphere of work can affect our professional work. Principle 9 (GDC, 2013) is explicit about this when it states: 'Make sure your personal behaviour maintains patients' confidence in you and the dental profession'.

Because the dental profession constitutes a readily identifiable group, many kinds of misconduct by the few can lead to bad consequences for the many. One person's misconduct or lack of character hurts his or her fellow professionals. Interestingly, this observation insists directly only on good image and not on genuine goodness. A dental professional may be motivated to appear to be a good person because they deem it good for business. Inside, they may feel quite differently, they may even act differently should the opportunity arise. In this age of social media, it becomes more difficult to be a Jekyll and Hyde.

Professionalism encompasses behaviours, that is, what we do that demonstrates we are professionals, but probably even more important than behaviours are attitudes, values and beliefs. If those foundations are shaky then the behaviours exhibited will be at best insincere, at worst bad. You can fake an expected behaviour for a while but eventually your underlying values and beliefs will show through. It's interesting that many companies are now recruiting staff for their values and beliefs rather than skills. The thinking is that you can teach skills but if the values and beliefs are in conflict with those of the company then you cannot change those. The method is known as values-based recruitment (VBR). There has been some introduction of this into dental student recruitment. Health Education England (HEE) (2106) has stated that VBR is a priority. The mandate to HEE from the government requires that:

'HEE will oversee delivery of a national values based recruitment framework and associated tools and resources by October 2014 and ensure that selection into all new NHS funded training posts incorporates testing of values based recruitment by March 2015.' (p. 25)

The values that the NHS promotes are included in the NHS Constitution (Department of Health, 2015) and it is expected that all NHS employees will demonstrate these values, which are:

- working together for patients
- respect and dignity
- commitment to quality of care
- compassion
- improving lives
- everyone counts.

What does professionalism encompass?

As dental professionals, we are not only concerned with our own behaviour. We are in service to our patients, we put their interests before our own. We have a duty to not only respect the rights of our patients but also to undertake actions that allow those rights to be enacted. What do I mean by this? If our patients have a right to expect confidentiality (which they do) then we have a duty to undertake actions that will ensure confidentiality is maintained. All rights are twinned with duties.

How should a professional behave?

When I ask this in presentations, the frequent answer is – with professionalism. While this is clearly a 'tongue in cheek' response, it does underline the fact that how a professional should behave is not an easy thing to get to grips with. Perhaps the more difficult aspect is – when should a professional behave? Now it's my turn to be 'tongue in cheek'. There is a simple response to this and a more complex one. The simple one first – all the time! I'm going to expand on both these aspects. How to behave first. Being a professional and behaving as a professional is character driven and those character traits are probably acquired and developed at a young age (see Chapter 2).

When to behave seems to be a difficult concept for some dental professionals to fully absorb. I wrote above that the way a professional behaves and demonstrates professionalism is character driven. It is innate and should be unconscious. If you have to think about it, you are probably faking it. You cannot behave in one way when at work and a different way when you are not at work. Let me give an example: you cannot be honest at work and dishonest outside work. You cannot act with integrity at work and without integrity outside work. We are complete individuals, our character cannot be contextual. Patients must be able to trust their dental professionals, which means all the time, not just whilst you are in the surgery. If you read GDC determinations, which are in the public domain on the GDC website, you sometimes come across cases where clearly the registrant thought what they do in their own time outside work should have no relevance to what they do at work. The phrase 'but I'm a good clinician' comes to mind.

An opinion piece by Afflick and Macnish (2016) gave me considerable pause for thought. They raised the issue of the reputation of the individual dental professional, the impact on the profession as a whole and links to fitness to practise. The piece made me think whether as dental professionals we just do a 'job', albeit a highly skilled job that involves considerable technical expertise, or are we 'professionals'? Being a professional working within a profession seems to me to embrace so much more than just the job and the clinical skills we use. The opinion piece brought into focus the difficulty of separating the performance of dentistry from the person performing it. It also highlighted how individuals act differently within work and outside work (at home and play).

This interests me from an ethical perspective. Is it possible for character traits to be switched on and off, to be context specific? In Chapter 6, I have analysed fitness to practise cases over a period of 3 years. A high proportion involve non-clinical aspects, largely behaviour that the GDC considered to be outside the attributes that a registrant deemed fit to practise should display. Often, it is these behaviours that figure prominently in the most serious determinations. An interesting question would be – does the profession as a whole agree with the standards that our regulatory body has set when judging behaviours? Even more interesting, would the population, the public, our patients, society, agree?

Afflick and Macnish discuss the role of character and its relationship to professions and professionals. Essentially, there is a direct link to virtue ethics and the assertion that professionals are virtuous people, that is, of good character. The point is made that with regard to the GDC, public opinion is an important consideration when deciding if a registrant's behaviour affects the reputation of the whole profession. As I state above, public opinion has not been tested and even if it is, it is likely to be a moveable feast changing over the years and thus perhaps not a reliable, consistent measure of character and reputation impact.

It is this aspect of professionalism that seems to be the most difficult for registrants to appreciate and maintain. Generally, dental professionals understand how they should act when working with patients, with a few exceptions. Understanding that this also applies when not working with patients and outside the surgery is more challenging.

Societal expectations of professionals

Whether it is right or wrong, society expects different behaviour from its professionals. We ignore this at our peril. Society confers benefits on those who are professionals and we have obligations to maintain in return for our status. Whilst this is almost certainly true, the concepts of what is a profession and professionalism are dynamic and their definition is not fixed.

Flexner (1915, p. 576) was the first to attempt to delineate the basic characteristics unique to a profession.

'... professional activity was basically intellectual, carrying with it great personal responsibility; it was learned, being based on great knowledge and not merely routine; it was practical, rather than academic or theoretic; its technique could be taught, this being the basis of professional education; it was strongly organized internally; and it was motivated by altruism, the professions viewing themselves as working for some aspect of the good of society.'

Carr-Saunders and Wilson (1933) show that professionalism as a model of how healthcare practitioners should behave is not particularly old. In the early 1930s, the characteristics attributed to professionals by society began to be explicitly described and more systematically analysed.

In 1972, Schein suggested eight characteristics of professionalism.

1. Full-time occupation
2. Strong motivation or calling for the career
3. Specialised body of knowledge and skills acquired during a prolonged period of education and training
4. Decision making on behalf of the client in terms of principles, theories and propositions
5. Service orientation
6. Service based on the objective needs of the client and mutual trust
7. Autonomy of judgement for performance
8. Formation of professional associations and other professional credentials

Over the past 45+ years, a number of these characteristics have stood the test of time and are still relevant. However, some are looking a little dated. For example, decision making on behalf of the client could be construed as paternalism, an ethical concept that has fallen from favour. Service orientation is another attribute that is undergoing changes as cosmetic procedures compete against 'health' interventions.

However, regardless of the evolution of professionalism as a concept, the character of dental professionals is still of considerable interest to patients and society.

Character

'One's character is one's fate.'

(Heraclitus, c.540–c.480 BC, Greek philosopher)

Character represents an interlocked set of personal values and virtues which normally guide conduct. Character is about who we are and who we become and includes, amongst other things, the virtues of responsibility, honesty, self-reliance, reliability, generosity, self-discipline and a sense of identity and purpose.

Taylor (2017) defines character as 'a set of personal traits or dispositions that produce specific moral emotions, inform motivation and guide conduct'. Miller (2013), a professor of philosophy and the director of the Character Project at Wake Forest University in North Carolina, defines someone's character as primarily consisting of character traits and the relationship between them. According to Miller, moral character traits fall into two broad categories: moral virtues and moral vices. Honesty and humility are examples of virtues, cruelty and cowardice are vices. 'Virtues are acquired excellences,' Miller says. 'We are not born with them, but it is possible to develop them slowly over time.'

A virtue has many features.

• It leads to good actions that are appropriate to the situation.
• It leads to actions that are performed in a variety of different situations relevant to the virtue.
• It leads to actions that are done for appropriate reasons or motives.
• It leads to a pattern of motivation and action that is stable and reliable over time.

For example, Miller explains that an honest person does the honest thing in relevant circumstances, which range widely to include the courtroom, a party, the office, etc. This is a stable feature of their character that persists over time. When they do the honest thing, they do it for the right reasons. Wanting to make a good impression or wanting to avoid guilt would not count as good motives or reasons, Miller says.

Aristotle, ancient Greek philosopher and the founder of character theory, is often referenced when speaking about morality and virtues. He viewed doing something against moral principles, compromising one's integrity, as more of a tragedy than a loss.

Building blocks of character

The Jubilee Centre for Character and Virtues at the University of Birmingham has undertaken considerable work into how character can be built, nurtured and grown. Its depiction of the building blocks of character is given in Figure 3.1. The four building blocks of intellectual virtue, moral virtue, performance virtue and civic virtue form the underpinning for practical wisdom or phronesis. Practical wisdom is an ability to act virtuously in an overarching way. This then leads to a flourishing individual and society.

Flourishing individuals and society

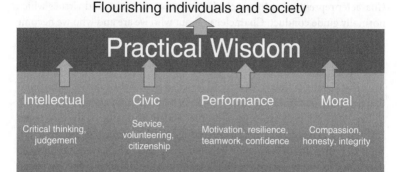

Figure 3.1 Building blocks of character.

The Jubilee Centre publishes widely on the subjects of character and virtues in both education and the professions. I recommend its research report on virtuous medical practice (Arthur *et al.*, 2015) which is available from its website.

Ethical frameworks within which professionals operate

Dental professionals are products of the society they operate within. For those born and raised in the UK, our ethical framework is acquired as we grow and mature. For those who move to the UK, the ethical framework can occasionally seem strange, unclear and difficult to get to grips with. However, everyone can usually 'sign up to' some ethical norms or core morality, for example;

- not to lie
- not to steal property
- to keep promises
- to respect the rights of others
- not to kill or cause harm to innocent people.

Sadly, not everyone in the population does observe these ethical norms. If they did, we would have little need for laws, prisons or a penal system.

Certain groups in society have specific ethical norms. For dental professionals, these are encapsulated in the standards and principles of the GDC.

- Put patients' interests first.
- Communicate effectively with patients.
- Obtain valid consent.
- Have a clear and effective complaints procedure.
- Maintain and protect patients' information.
- Work with colleagues in a way that is in patients' best interests.

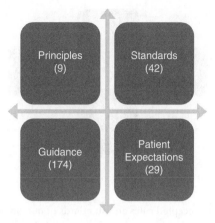

Figure 3.2 GDC standards for the dental team.

- Maintain, develop and work within your professional knowledge and skills.
- Raise concerns if patients are at risk.
- Make sure your personal behaviour maintains patients' confidence in you and the dental profession.

Alongside the nine principles there are:

- 42 standards: what registrants must do to ensure that patient expectations are met
- 29 patient expectations: what patients can expect from the dental team
- 174 pieces of guidance: how registrants meet the standards.

These are all equally important and supplemented by additional guidance (www.gdc-uk.org). The relationship of these four elements are depicted in figure 3.2.

How does character relate to professionalism?

The *Oxford English Reference Dictionary* defines character as:

1. *The collective qualities or characteristics (mental and moral) that distinguish a person or thing.*
2. *A moral strength.*

A characteristic is defined as some typical and distinctive feature. Let's look at the concept of 'moral' and drill down a little further.

'Moral' has the following definitions.

- Concerned with goodness or badness of human character or behaviour or the distinction between right and wrong.

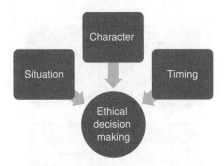

Figure 3.3 Components for ethical decision making.

- Concerned with accepted rules and standards of human behaviour.
- Conforming to accepted standards of general conduct.

Research by Gunia *et al.* (2014) suggests that character is only one dimension to consider; timing and situation can also affect whether a good ethical decision is made. It makes sense that individuals make better decisions and choices when they are fresh, at their most resilient and most able to exert self-control. Figure 3.3 is a visual image of bringing together the three dimensions to impact upon ethical decision making.

This adds complexity to consideration of fitness to practise that suggests that the context of ethical decisions made by an individual should be included alongside consideration of character traits. It also affects successful remediation.

Tests of integrity

Integrity is an important aspect of professional character. It is generally considered to be closely related to honesty and maintaining strong moral principles that the individual refuses to change, no matter what the temptation.

'*Have the courage to say no. Have the courage to face the truth. Do the right thing because it is right. These are the magic keys to living your life with integrity.*' (W. Clement Stone, 1902–2002)

Coleman (2009) suggests that a test of integrity is when we know the right thing to do, but it's hard to do for one reason or another, for example a strong sense of loyalty towards others. Other reasons why it may be difficult to do the right thing include the following.

- It will be unpopular.
- There is a lot of pressure not to do the right thing.
- Bribery, bullying, blackmail.
- There is a lot to gain from not doing the right thing, for example financial reward.

Dental professionals who are found to have committed fraud or theft or exploitation of patients for their own gain can be deemed to have failed tests of their integrity.

Virtue ethics

Virtue ethics is concerned with the person rather than the action. The underlying premise is that a virtuous person will always choose to do the right thing for the right reasons. The virtuous person does not need to be told what is right – it flows from their inner virtue and character.

From an ethical and moral point of view, dental professionals can be considered to be virtuous individuals. Aristotle, the Greek philosopher of ancient times, is considered to be the 'father' of virtue ethics. For Aristotle, a virtue is a trait of a person's character (*hexis*); once developed, it is a stable trait that influences the way a person acts from a moral point of view.

Unlike other ethical philosophies, virtue ethics tells us how we should *be* rather than how we should *act* and that underpins our character, our values and how we interact with others. Examples of virtues are benevolence (doing good), compassion (an awareness of the distress of others with the desire to alleviate it) and honesty (not lying or cheating, being truthful and sincere). Our character and the traits we display are integral to ourselves, not something we can turn on or off depending on the situation we find ourselves in. It is almost impossible to have a sincere and authentic situational character. A situational character is when an individual displays one set of character traits and virtues in one situation, perhaps at work, and another in another situation, perhaps at home.

It is for this reason that I believe the character and virtues we display outside the working environment directly affect our working persona. Dental professionals cannot display poor character traits outside work (for example, being dishonest) and not expect that to reflect on their professional life. A person is who and what they are, wholly and totally, they cannot be dishonest between 5pm and 8am and then honest between 8am and 5pm and remain authentic, particularly if they are a professional. The trust of patients is embedded in their trust of our character, attitudes and behaviour.

The important message is that poor behaviour outside the working day, outside the surgery, can lead to a complaint or a fitness to practise investigation and the quality of the professional's clinical expertise will be largely irrelevant. Skill is not a character trait. A person with a bad character could be a very skilful person.

The central focus for virtue ethics is character – how should I be? Which replaces – what should I do? Virtue is a trait or quality deemed to be morally good. The opposite of virtue is vice. The goal is to seek excellence of

character – the virtues. It is difficult and needs practice. For every character trait, there is a continuum from excess to deficit, and neither end of the
continuum is desirable.

Excess	Virtue	Deficit
Rashness ←	Courage	→ Cowardice
Profligacy ←	Generosity	→ Meanness

However, virtue ethics is not good at telling us how to act, only that we should
do what the ideally virtuous person would do. In addition, there is insufficient
guidance on how we deal with dilemmas.

A virtue is the 'sweet spot' between excess and deficiency, sometimes
referred to as 'the golden mean'.

Aristotle believed that being a virtuous person required practice and
experience, so that a person developed wisdom and increased their ability to
be virtuous. To me, this means that a dental professional grows into virtues.
It also seems that a person may act with either excess or deficit of a virtue
before developing 'the golden mean'. I feel this is very important when dealing
with lapses in professionalism and it has a serious message for remediation.
By that, I mean a person can learn from lapses in virtuous behaviour and
learn to become more virtuous. Character traits are not either present or
absent but can be improved and developed. I suspect that the presence of
reflection and a heightened sense of insight would aid the process.

Honesty and dishonesty

'To be honest is to be real, genuine, and bona fide. To be dishonest is to
be partly feigned, forged, fake, or fictitious. Honesty expresses both self-
respect and respect for others. Dishonesty fully respects neither oneself
nor others. Honesty imbues lives with openness, reliability and candour;
it expresses a disposition to live in the light. Dishonesty seeks shade,
cover, or concealment. It is a disposition to live partly in the dark'

(Bennett, 1993, p. 599)

Honesty is a virtue and dishonesty a vice. It might appear as if this is an
either/or situation – a person is either honest or dishonest – but that assump-
tion is simplistic and unlikely to be correct. All individuals will display both
honesty and dishonesty at times during their life. There is a continuum with
100% honesty at one end and 100% dishonesty at the other. At most times in
our lives and in the decisions we choose to make, we operate somewhere
along that continuum. Whether you consider an act to be dishonest may be

affected by your upbringing and the values that became instilled in you from a young age. Other factors that will affect the ethical choices you make include the environment, the context of the act, peers and friends. Perhaps even our physical condition can affect our ethical decisions. When we are tired or under pressure, energy levels fall and it can be harder to act ethically. Temptations to act with poor judgement and make unethical decisions rise and are more difficult to resist.

Some interesting research undertaken by Gunia *et al.* (2014) shows an even more subtle influence on when during the day people are more likely to display honesty or dishonesty – our chronotype. Chronotype describes whether we are at our best in the morning or the evening. The research suggested that people who are considered to be 'morning people' or 'larks' are at their most honest in the morning and become less so as the day progresses. The reverse appears to be true for 'night owls' who are at their most honest in the evening and less so earlier in the day. Professor Christopher Barnes noted: 'There is mounting evidence that "good" people can be unethical and "bad" people can be ethical depending on the pressures of the moment' (Gunia *et al.*, 2014).

This research opens a fascinating debate on whether the continuum of virtue or vice may be more dependent on the environment and the pressures placed upon individuals than was thought to be the case.

Nelsonian dishonesty

The principle of Nelsonian dishonesty is described in the case of Twinsectra Ltd v Yardley and others [2002] UKHL 12. This principle is derived from when Lord Nelson, at the Battle of Copenhagen, made a deliberate decision to place the telescope to his blind eye in order to avoid seeing what he knew he would see if he placed it to his good eye. As dental registrants, we cannot apply Nelsonian dishonesty. If we know a colleague has acted in a way that is against the professional standards or rules or where their behaviour or health places patient safety at risk, we must do something. If we do not, then our own registration is at risk.

The importance of honesty and integrity for regulated professionals was reinforced by High Court judgements on cases submitted by the Professional Standards Authority (PSA) (annual report 2015/16). The PSA noted the seriousness with whwich fitness to practise panels regarded dishonesty and also the level of sanctions applied.

The GDC Guidance for the Practice Committees (2016) has the following to say about dishonesty.

'Patients, employers, colleagues and others have a right to rely on registrants' integrity. Important choices about treatment options and

significant financial decisions can be made on the basis not only of registrants' skill but also of their honesty. Dishonesty, particularly when associated with professional practice, is highly damaging to a registrant's fitness to practise and to public confidence in dental professionals.'

The issue of dishonesty and dishonest behaviour cuts to the heart of public perceptions of integrity, not least because patients and service users are, by definition, vulnerable. The PSA (2016) commissioned research to understand the views of the public and health and care professionals across the UK on how different types and degrees of dishonest behaviour are seen to influence fitness to practise and professionalism in different contexts and in a range of health and care professions.

Nine scenarios were considered in the research, involving:

- dishonesty in relation to patient records
- dishonesty in relation to qualifications or employment history
- dishonesty in relation to registration status or indemnity insurance
- dishonesty in relation to working at another job
- dishonesty (tax fraud) outside the immediate context of professional practice
- dishonesty in relation to convictions or previous identity
- dishonesty in relation to patient interactions
- lying about relationships with colleagues or patients to conceal inappropriate practice
- theft from patients or colleagues.

There was a consensus that premeditated, systematic or long-standing abuse of professional trust or dishonesty in the context of financial gain or sexual exploitation should be grounds for rapid deregistration.

The majority, however, with the exception of the most egregious cases, took a pragmatic and tolerant view on the appropriate disposals for dishonesty in fitness to practise cases. The tendency was towards an emphasis on behaviour change and learning and rehabilitative and constructive outcomes, which allowed registrants to continue in the profession. This was particularly the case where individuals showed insight and remorse and seemed willing to change their behaviour.

The PSA also commissioned work by the University of Surrey and Royal Holloway University of London (Gallagher and Jago, 2016) to review cases involving dishonesty from the PSA database of final fitness to practise outcomes, and to develop a typology of different kinds of dishonest misconduct. The study identified six types of dishonesty. Professional and private life was differentiated where applicable.

- Dishonesty by omission: not disclosing, where the truth is withheld.
- Dishonesty by commission: lying, where a registrant tells an untruth.

- Impersonation: assuming the identity of another person.
- Theft: stealing.
- Fraud: deceiving.
- Academic dishonesty: cheating.

Of the 151 cases reviewed in the study, the three most common kinds of dishonest activities were:

- failure to disclose convictions/cautions to the regulator either upon registration or for the purposes of retention on the register (19 cases)
- simple theft of identified monies, prescription pads and medication or drug paraphernalia (18 cases)
- receiving sick pay and salary from a second employer simultaneously (13 cases).

There is no statutory definition of what dishonesty means in criminal law. This means that there is room for interpretation. What has developed is a two-stage test.

1. Was the individual's conduct dishonest according to the standards of the ordinary reasonable or decent person?

If the answer to this question was 'yes', then:

2. Did the individual realise that the ordinary reasonable or decent person would regard his/her conduct as dishonest?

This is now the common law test for dishonesty, which is used in all legal proceedings where dishonesty is alleged.

An aspect relating to cases of dishonesty is the ability (or perceived ability) to remediate. It seems that the GDC fitness to practise panels take a position that dishonest conduct is behaviour related to character and as such is difficult to remedy. A number of factors will affect the ability to remediate, including the degree of dishonesty, the length of time over which it was conducted and the internal and external factors acting on the individual at the time. However, perhaps the most important factor is the effect dishonesty of a professional has on the overall reputation of the profession and the perception of the public and patients. Dental professionals occupy a position of privilege and trust in society and must make sure that their conduct at all times justifies both their patients' and the public's trust in the profession.

Arthur (2009) makes an interesting observation.

> 'Integrity and particularly honesty are rather old-fashioned virtues but are seen as important. This may be a relic of the time when "character" was partly synonymous with "reputation" and, at least for the lower orders, "honest" was partly synonymous with "of good character".
> Whether this is partly responsible for the words rolling off the tongues of participants, these old-fashioned virtues seem to be part of at least some modern ideas of what it is to be a good person.'

Perhaps it is time for a rethink on the ability to remediate character flaws and on society's perception of whether a remediated professional affects the reputation of the profession as a whole.

'The ultimate measure of a man is not where he stands in moments of comfort and convenience, but where he stands at times of challenge and controversy.'

(Martin Luther King Jr, 1968, last speech)

Communication

There are whole libraries of books, articles and training programmes on communication. It is one of the nine principles of the GDC: 'Communicate effectively with patients'. Clearly it is important when working with patients, colleagues and staff to communicate well, and yet issues of communication figure highly in GDC fitness to practise hearings.

Good communication usually begins with rapport, being able to develop an affinity between two people so that they trust one another. Rapport with patients is essential to the therapeutic relationship and rapport with colleagues and staff is essential for good team working. The greater the rapport, the more influence can follow. For dental professionals, being able to influence patients to take responsibility for their oral health is important. When a patient trusts their dental professional, they are more likely to actively engage in their own care. Patients are rarely able to assess their own dental treatment, but what they are fully qualified to judge is the level of communication that passes between themselves and their dental professional. It is generally accepted that a superb clinician with poor communication skills is more likely to generate a complaint than a passable clinician with excellent communication skills.

Mehrabian (1981) details the importance of verbal and non-verbal communication as demonstrated in Figure 3.4. Communication is a combination of what is said, what is seen and what is heard. This makes it very easy for miscommunication to occur. In addition, the words we use are the smallest factor in communication. Whilst that might be helpful from a language point of view, it makes the interpretation of communication much more difficult. That's because the non-verbal part of communication can mean different things to different people. This can also apply to the stress placed on words, our speech rate and volume. In a multicultural profession, providing services for multicultural patient groups, miscommunication and misinterpretation are very likely to happen. An important part of Mehrabian's work was the interaction between the three aspects of communication. When there is a mismatch between the words that are spoken and the non-verbal signs (the

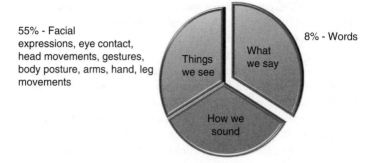

55% - Facial
expressions, eye contact,
head movements, gestures,
body posture, arms, hand, leg
movements

8% - Words

Things
we see

What
we say

How we
sound

37% - Rate, volume, pitch, fluency

Figure 3.4 How we communicate. Source: A Mehrabian (1981)

body language) demonstrated, the person receiving the communication will give more weight to the body language than to the words.

Chapter 8 covers tools that can help to understand the underpinning of good communication.

Criminal record, convictions and cautions

Every year there are a number of fitness to practise referrals involving convictions and/or cautions. As part of their process, the police will inform regulatory bodies when a conviction or caution has been given to an individual. The GDC when informed in this way will open a fitness to practise investigation. All registrants are required to inform the GDC as soon as a conviction or caution has been received. If they do not, then non-co-operation with the regulator will compound the issue.

If a registrant has a positive criminal record check for assault, theft or minor drug offences then this may make it difficult for them to find employment. Generally, convictions become spent after a period of time, for example after 10 years from conviction for someone who has been sentenced to prison for between 6 and 30 months.

Since 2003, all dentists, dental hygienists and dental therapists have been required to declare criminal convictions and/or cautions when registering with the GDC and since 14 May 2009, clinical dental technicians, dental nurses, dental technicians and orthodontic therapists have been required to do the same. As of 29 May 2013, applicants have not been required to declare protected convictions and cautions. Notifications of criminality may also be received through third parties and the Notifiable Occupations Scheme, which is operated by the police.

In 2013 the GDC published new guidance which requires all registrants to inform the GDC if on, or after, 30 September 2013 they:

- are charged with a criminal offence
- are found guilty of a criminal offence
- receive a conditional discharge for an offence
- accept a criminal caution (including a conditional caution), or otherwise formally admit to committing a criminal offence
- accept the option of paying a penalty notice for a disorder offence (in England and Wales), a penalty notice under the Justice Act (Northern Ireland) 2011 or a fixed penalty notice under the Antisocial Behaviour etc. (Scotland) Act 2004
- receive a formal adult warning in Scotland.

Registrants do not need to inform the GDC of the following:

- a fixed penalty notice for a road traffic offence
- a fixed penalty notice issued by local authorities (for example, for offences such as dog fouling or graffiti)
- an antisocial behaviour, preventive justice or other social order.

For existing registrants, both self-referred and third party referred, cautions and convictions will be processed by the fitness to practise department. For third-party referrals, consideration will also be given to whether any misconduct arises from the registrant's failure to notify the GDC of the offence or if a false declaration was made by the registrant on their application.

Cautions

In England and Wales, a caution may be given by the police when there is sufficient evidence for a conviction but it is not considered to be in the public interest to pursue criminal proceedings. The registrant must have admitted guilt and consented to a caution in order to be given one. A dental professional who accepts a caution must inform the GDC immediately. The GDC will decide if the caution currently impairs the registrant's fitness to practise and therefore should be investigated.

Conditional discharges

A conditional discharge can only be imposed after a person has been found guilty. It must, however, be reported to the GDC by the registrant. However, it is not a conviction, so the GDC cannot treat it in the same way as a caution or a conviction. This means that the GDC must decide if the reasons that led to the conditional discharge would lead to an allegation of misconduct and if the registrant's fitness to practise is impaired.

Scotland

In Scotland, the Procurator Fiscal may decide that prosecuting an alleged offence is not in the public interest and may apply an alternative measure. Alternatives to prosecution include a warning, a fiscal fine, a compensation order, a work order, a road traffic fixed penalty or rehabilitative support. Acceptance of the offer of an alternative to prosecution does not, unlike a caution, amount to an admission of guilt by the accused. Because of this, the Professional Conduct Committee (PCC) is not able to treat a Scottish alternative to prosecution as though it were a caution or conviction, and thus a means by which a registrant's fitness to practise may be impaired under the Act. Rather, where an offer of an alternative to prosecution has been accepted, the PCC must consider whether the events that led to the offer and acceptance of an alternative to prosecution amount to misconduct, such that the registrant's fitness to practise is impaired (French, 2017).

Protected conviction or caution

Certain convictions and cautions have 'protected' status. For convictions, this is defined as follows.
- It is not a 'listed offence'. A listed offence is defined in paragraph 5 of article 2A in the 2013 Order AND
- No custodial sentence (or service detention) was imposed AND
- The individual has no other convictions AND
- It was received by a person aged under 18 at the time of the conviction and 5 years and 6 months or more have elapsed OR
- It was received by a person aged 18 or over at the time of the conviction and 11 years or more have elapsed.

For cautions to be protected, the following must apply.
- It is not a listed offence AND
- It was given to a person aged under 18 at the time of the caution and 2 years or more have elapsed OR
- It was given to a person aged 18 years or over at the time of the caution and 6 years or more have elapsed.

Registrants and those applying for registration or restoration are required to declare all convictions and cautions that are not considered 'protected'.

Protected status for convictions that are not 'listed' offences is only applicable to those aged between 24.5 years and 29 years, depending on whether they were either under 18 or over 18 when they received the conviction. Protected status for cautions extends to those aged between 20 and 26 years of age, again depending on whether they were under 18 or over 18 when they received the caution. For those older than 30, protected status does not apply to convictions or cautions.

The Rehabilitation of Offenders Act 1974 allows for convictions to have a time limit for disclosure. This does not apply to healthcare professionals. For all dental professionals, all cautions and convictions need to be disclosed, and are included in DBS criminal records check.

References

Afflick, P. and Macnish, K. (2016) Should 'fitness to practise' include safeguarding the reputation of the profession? *British Dental Journal*, **221**, 545–546.

Arthur, J. (2009) *Graduates of Character. Values and Character: Higher Education and Graduate Employment*. Jubilee Centre, University of Birmingham.

Arthur, J., Kristjansson, K., Thomas, H. *et al.* (2015) *Virtuous Medical Practice*. Research Report. Jubilee Centre, University of Birmingham.

Bennett, W.J. (ed.) (1993) *The Book of Virtues: A Treasury of Great Moral Stories*. Simon and Schuster, New York.

Carr-Saunders, A.M. and Wilson, P.A. (1933) *The Professions*. Reprinted by the Clarendon Press, Oxford, 1984.

Coleman, S. (2009) The problems of duty and loyalty. *Journal of Military Ethics*, **8**(2), 105–115.

Cooke, S., Badini, L. and Jones, D. (2013) Autonomy, in *Accountability and Professional Behaviour in Teaching, Medicine and Law*. Centre for Character and Values, University of Birmingham.

Dental Board of the United Kingdom (1957) *Minutes with Reports of Committees, etc. for the Year 1956 and General Index to the Minutes 1921–1956*. Vol. **XV**.

Department of Health (2015) *The NHS Constitution for England: Guidelines*. Available at: www.gov.uk

Flexner, A. (1915) Is social work a profession? *Social Welfare History Project*. Available at: http://socialwelfare.library.vcu.edu/social-work/is-social-work-a-profession-1915/ (accessed 11 January 2018).

French, J. (2017) *Guidance for Decision Makers on the Impact of Convictions and Cautions, v.2.2*. General Dental Council, London.

Gallagher, A. and Jago, R. (2016) *A Typology of Dishonesty. Illustrations from the Professional Standards Authority Section 29 Database*. Royal Holloway, University of London.

General Dental Council (GDC) (2013) *Standards for the Dental Team*. General Dental Council, London.

General Dental Council (2016) *Guidance for the Practice Committees including Indicative Sanction Guidance*. General Dental Council, London.

Gunia, B., Barnes, C.M. and Sah, S. (2014) The morality of larks and owls: unethical behavior depends on chronotype as well as time-of-day. *Psychological Science*, **25**, 2272–2274.

Health Education England (2016) *Values Based Recruitment Framework*. Health Education England, Taunton.

King, M.L. Jr (1948) *The Purpose of Education*. Morehouse College, Atlanta.

Mehrabian, A. (1981) *Silent Messages: Implicit Communication of Emotions and Attitudes.* Wadsworth, Belmont.

Miller, C. (2013) *Moral Character: An Empirical Theory.* Oxford University Press, Oxford.

Professional Standards Authority (2016) Annual report 2014/15. Professional Standards Authority, London, p. 15.

Schein, E.H. (1972) *Professional Education.* McGraw-Hill, New York.

Taylor, J. (2017) *Character education, what is it and can it really be taught?* Powerpoint presentation, University of Warwick.

Further Reading

Barnes, C.M., Schaubroeck, J.M., Huth, M. and Ghumman, S., (2011) Lack of sleep and unethical behaviour. *Organizational Behavior and Human Decision Processes,* **115**, 169–180.

Health Education England (2014) *Values Based Recruitment. A Survey of Existing Recruitment to NHS Funded Undergraduate Training Programmes.*

Chapter 4 **Regulation of dentistry and dental professionals**

In Chapter 2, we considered how issues of poor performance can arise and the factors that contribute to and underpin poor performance. Then the building blocks and components of professionalism were covered in Chapter 3. In this chapter, I will look at the regulation of dentistry and dental professionals. This will include the organisations that play key roles in the UK. It is also important to ask why regulation is necessary and what is 'right touch' regulation?

Regulation of dentistry and dental professionals in the UK is not straightforward; a number of organisations are involved and they can be different between the countries of the UK.

Before looking at each of these organisations and the role they play, I would first like to consider what regulation is and why it is required.

Regulation

1. *General*: principle or rule (with or without the coercive power of law) employed in controlling, directing, or managing an activity, organization or system.
2. *Law*: rule, based on and meant to carry out a specific piece of legislation (such as for the protection of the environment). Regulations are enforced usually by a regulatory agency formed or mandated to carry out the purpose or provisions of a legislation. Also called regulatory requirement.

Source: www.businessdictionary.com/definition/regulation.html

This definition makes it clear that regulation is not something to be taken lightly. An organisation that enforces regulation is a powerful one.

Dentistry is a regulated profession and dental services, that is the care and treatment provided by dental professionals to their patients, are regulated services.

Regulation of healthcare professionals primarily exists to protect public safety. The object of the regulation is the individual professional.

How to Survive Dental Performance Difficulties, First Edition. Janine Brooks.
© 2018 John Wiley & Sons Ltd. Published 2018 by John Wiley & Sons Ltd.

Regulation of individual professionals began in the UK with the establishment of the GMC in 1858. The organisations and systems of healthcare are also regulated, generally by different regulators. However, four of the nine healthcare regulators have a dual role that includes individuals and also a degree of jurisdiction over businesses engaged in that profession. The GDC is one of those four and, for example, it has requirements relevant to directors of dental bodies as given in section 34 of the Dentists Act 1984.

Each healthcare regulatory body has the same overarching functions.

- Setting the standards of behaviour, competence and education that professionals must meet.
- Dealing with concerns from patients, the public and others about professionals who are unfit to practise because of poor health, misconduct or poor performance.
- Keeping registers of professionals who are fit to practise and setting the requirements for periodic re-registration (and in some cases revalidation) for each profession.

When the GDC was originally set up, it had a more expanded role to include research, loans to students and dental health education of the public (Dental Board, 1957) but over the years these additional roles have been lost.

Having briefly considered regulation and why it is needed in healthcare, the next section reviews the role of the bodies involved in healthcare regulation. Initially, I have summarised the roles undertaken by the GMC, the General Pharmaceutical Council and the GDC in regulation.

General Medical Council

The General Medical Council (GMC) is the professional regulator of doctors. Prior to 1956, it also regulated dentists (only) through a subcommittee, the Dental Board. It provides guidance and standards and investigates complaints against doctors.

1. To practise safely, doctors must be competent in what they do. They must establish and maintain effective relationships with patients, respect patients' autonomy and act responsibly and appropriately if they or a colleague fall ill and their performance suffers.
2. But these attributes, while essential, are not enough. Doctors have a respected position in society and their work gives them privileged access to patients, some of whom may be very vulnerable. A doctor whose conduct has shown that he cannot justify the trust placed in him should not continue in unrestricted practice while that remains the case.

3. In short, the public is entitled to expect that their doctor is fit to practise, and follows our principles of good practice described in Good Medical Practice. It sets out the standards of competence, care and conduct expected of doctors. (www.gmc-uk.org, published April 2014, Code: GMC/MFTP/0414)

General Pharmaceutical Council

The General Pharmaceutical Council (GPC) is the professional regulator for pharmacists, pharmacy technicians and pharmacy premises. It was established via the Pharmacy Order 2010 and operates throughout Great Britain, (England, Wales and Scotland).

'We consider a pharmacy professional fit to practise when they can demonstrate the skills, knowledge, character and health required to do their job safely and effectively.

We describe fitness to practise as a person's suitability to be on the register without restrictions. In practical terms, this means: maintaining appropriate standards of proficiency ensuring you are of good health and good character, and you are adhering to principles of good practice set out in our various, standards, guidance and advice.'

(General Pharmaceutical Council, www.pharmacyregulation.org)

General Dental Council

The GDC is the professional regulatory body for all categories of dental professional in the UK. It has been the regulator of dental professionals since it gained independence from the GMC in 1956, a transition that is noted by Sir Wilfred Fish as taking 10 years to achieve. It is regulated and overseen by the Professional Standards Authority, as are all the nine healthcare regulators.

You cannot work as a dental professional in the UK unless you are registered with the GDC. Those who attempt to work in dentistry without registration are breaking the law. Each dental registrant pays an annual retention fee (ARF) to the GDC which permits them to be registered and to practise dentistry within their scope of practice depending on their registrant category.The GDC maintains the register and each dental professional is allocated a registrant number when they first register and they retain that number throughout their dental career until they retire and remove themselves from the register or they are erased by the GDC. Initial application to the GDC register is prescribed and the criteria can be found on the GDC website. The regulator's requirements include maintaining professional skills, knowledge checks and being of good character.

The overarching role and purpose of the GDC is to 'protect patients'. The organisation has statutory powers that it uses to fulfil its role, which is to:

- permit registration of those who satisfy requirements of education and training, health and good character
- set criteria and quality assure dental pre-registration education and training
- set standards of conduct, performance and ethics for the dental team
- investigate allegations of 'impaired fitness to practise' and take appropriate action
- protect the public from individuals carrying out dentistry while not registered
- require dental professionals to keep their skills up to date through criteria for continuing professional development (CPD) requirements.

The GDC introduced a new process of dealing with concerns in 2016, with the aim of encouraging resolution between the dental professional and the patient at a local level. It is known as GDC NHS Concerns Handling. The new process will deal with low-level concerns including:

- single, isolated incidents where there is not a pattern of repeated behaviour
- evidence of poor communication between the dental professional and the patient
- evidence of poor record keeping
- where the dental professional has failed to adequately explain dental charges.

It is hoped that the process will encourage an early conversation between the NHS and the patient to enable a more adequate assessment of which is the most appropriate organisation to investigate the concern.

Registration

To join the dental register, an individual must have attained specific qualifications. In some instances, an assessment is also necessary. The applicant must show that they have one of the following (current at October 2017):

- a recognised UK qualification
- a recognised European qualification
- a recognised non-European qualification
- an assessment of suitability to register, via a GDC panel assessment of skills and knowledge (in the case of non-European qualified persons with exempt person status)
- success in passing the Overseas Registration Exam (for non-European overseas-qualified dentists who do not benefit from enforceable community rights).

Following the UK's departure from the European Union, these criteria are likely to change in relation to dental professionals with a recognised European qualification, but the details are yet to emerge.

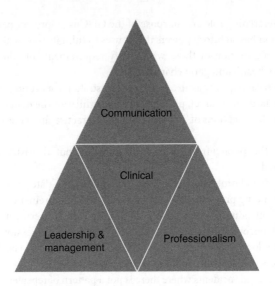

Figure 4.1 GDC learning outcome domains.

Non-dentist dental professionals who have an overseas qualification from outside the European Economic Area (EEA) can apply to the GDC for an assessment. The process takes approximately 4 months and at the end of 2017, there was no fee for the assessment. It is undertaken by the GDC registration assessment panel and if successful, the dental care professional is eligible to apply for registration with the GDC and may work in the UK.

All three regulators above refer to standards that they expect their registrants to demonstrate and adhere to if they are to be deemed fit to practise in that profession.

In the document *Preparing for Practice* (2012), the GDC describes the learning outcomes required for registration. Four domains are described that define the knowledge, skills, attitudes and behaviour that all registrants need to demonstrate at registration (Figure 4.1).

NHS England

NHS England (NHSE) commissions primary care services, including all dental services. The organisation oversees and manages dentists, doctors and optometrists who are registered on the NHS England National Performers List. There are national lists for medical, dental and ophthalmic performers. The lists provide an extra layer of reassurance for the public that GPs, dentists and opticians practising in the NHS are suitably qualified, have up-to-date training and appropriate English language skills and have passed other relevant checks such as with the Disclosure and Barring Service and the NHS Resolve (previously the NHS Litigation Authority). Primary Care Support England (PCSE) is responsible for administering entry and status changes to performers lists on behalf of NHSE. The decision to admit or decline an applicant to the national performers lists is the responsibility of NHSE.

There are two groups within NHSE that are concerned with performance of those on the national performers list: performers lists decision panels (PLDPs) and the performance advisory group (PAG). The PAGs investigate and advise while the PLDPs make decisions under the performers lists regulations. PAGs are present in each area team and consider complaints or concerns raised about dentists. They can investigate the issues and give advice. They report to PLDPs which are also present in each area team and decide on any action needed for individual performance cases that have been reviewed by the PAG. They can refer onwards to the GDC or the police or request an alert to be raised. They can also agree a remediation plan for a dental practitioner.

In Wales, the performers list is managed for NHS Wales by the Shared Services Partnership. In Scotland, the performers lists are managed by the health boards.

Care Quality Commission

The Care Quality Commission (CQC) is the regulator of health and social care in England. Dental providers are included in the CQC's remit.

All providers of regulated health and social care services have a legal responsibility to make sure they are meeting essential standards of quality and safety. The essential standards that the CQC uses to inspect services are described in the Health and Social Care Act 2008 (Regulated Activities) Regulations 2010 and the Care Quality Commission (Registration) Regulations 2009.

The CQC undertakes inspections of dental providers, including practices, community dental services, hospitals, corporate bodies, social enterprises and dental services in prisons on a regular basis. Its findings are published on its website and are within the public domain.

There are 16 essential standards that the CQC uses as the basis of its inspections.

- Respecting and involving people who use services
- Consent to care and treatment
- Care and welfare of people who use services
- Meeting nutritional needs
- Cooperating with other providers
- Safeguarding people who use services from abuse

- Cleanliness and infection control
- Management of medicines
- Safety and suitability of premises
- Safety, availability and suitability of equipment
- Requirements relating to workers
- Staffing
- Supporting staff
- Assessing and monitoring the quality of service provision
- Complaints
- Records (CQC, 2010)

Healthcare Inspectorate Wales

The Healthcare Inspectorate Wales (HIW) regulates and inspects NHS services and independent healthcare providers in Wales. This includes NHS dentists, dentists who undertake private work and dentists who provide a mixture of private and NHS work. The legal underpinning for HIW can be found in the Private Dentistry (Wales) Regulation 2008 and the Private Dentistry (Wales) (Amendment) Regulations. Its objectives are to assure quality, safety and effectiveness and it will also make recommendations for improvement. At an inspection, the following aspects of service delivery are reviewed.

- Patient experience: asking patients what they think about the practice.
- Standards: examining how the practice is meeting required standards relating to specific areas of dentistry.
- Management and leadership: how the practice is run. Checking that there are relevant policies and procedures to ensure that staff and patients are safe.
- Practice environment: looking at the building and facilities at the practice to check that it is fit for purpose and safe for patients and staff.

Each dental practice is inspected once every 3 years as a minimum. However, this can be more frequent if problems are brought to its attention.

Scotland

In Scotland, government-funded healthcare is administered by NHS National Services Scotland (NSS) and NHS Scotland. The work undertaken by NHS England (in England) is undertaken by the health boards and dentistry under the NHS and is managed by the Practitioner Services Division (PSD).

Payments under the NHS are made to dentists by the PSD on behalf of the health boards which are also responsible for running the Dental Reference Service (DRS). Dental Reference Officers (DRO) in Scotland are responsible for examining patients both in respect of dentists seeking prior approval for treatment, and for assessing the standard of the completed treatment, as well as verifying claims. The present DRS system for case assessment is currently being reviewed (October 2017).

The PSD has a clinical governance function and may ask dentists to send in record cards which are then checked against claim forms to corroborate claims which have been made for those patients. This check may also be performed in conjunction with a DRO patient examination.

There still exists an NHS disciplinary system in Scotland where a dentist's health board may refer a matter for investigation to a neighbouring health board if it believes a dentist may be in breach of their NHS terms of service.

The health boards maintain lists of dental practitioners.

Northern Ireland

Regulation and Quality Improvement Authority

The Regulation and Quality Improvement Authority (RQIA) is the independent regulatory body for Northern Ireland. Dentists who provide private dental care and treatment in Northern Ireland must be registered with the RQIA. The authority has a programme of inspections and reviews by which it monitors the quality of services. The role of the RQIA is to improve care, inform the population of their rights and influence policy with regard to the NHS in Northern Ireland.

Dentists who provide solely NHS care are not required to be registered with the RQIA.

Dental practices that do need to be registered must demonstrate that they are meeting appropriate general standards of quality and safety in all regulated activities.

Health and Social Care Board (HSCB)

The Health and Social Care (Disciplinary Procedures) Regulations (Northern Ireland) 2016 currently govern disciplinary proceedings in relation to some family health practitioners, including dentists. The Reference Committee initially considers serious disciplinary matters relating to dentists and may take one of the following actions.

- Take no action.
- Refer the matter to a tribunal.
- Refer the matter to the GDC.
- Refer the matter to the Police Service of Northern Ireland.

If the Reference Committee decides that a matter should be investigated, it will be referred to the Disciplinary Committee for consideration and decision. The role of the Disciplinary Committee is to undertake the HSCB's functions as appropriate under the Health and Personal Social Services

(Disciplinary Procedures) Regulations (Northern Ireland) 2016 with respect to disciplinary matters for dentists referred to it by the Reference Committee.

The Disciplinary Committee is composed of a legally qualified chairman, a lay person and, in dental cases, a dentist.

The Health and Personal Social Services (Disciplinary Procedures) Regulations 1996 currently govern disciplinary proceedings in relation to family health practitioners, including dentists. When the HSCB receives information which it considers could amount to an allegation that a practitioner has failed to comply with his or her terms of service, the Board can decide to:

• take no action
• refer the matter to a dental discipline committee
• refer the matter to the Health and Social Care Tribunal
• refer the matter to the General Dental Council
• refer the matter to the Police Service of Northern Ireland.

The above decision-making process will normally involve an initial consideration of the matter by a Board Investigating Officer, following which, if concerns remain, the matter will then be referred onto the Regional Professional Panel and, if appropriate, after consideration by that panel, further referred on to the Reference Committee which will make a final decision on whether the above steps are to be taken.

Professional Standards Authority

The Professional Standards Authority for Health and Social Care (PSA) was established on 1 December 2012, although its predecessor organisation was initially established in 2002. Its role and duties are set out in the Health and Social Care Act 2012. It is an independent UK-wide body and oversees nine healthcare regulators from whom it receives its primary funding (Table 4.1).

In brief, the PSA protects the public by raising standards of regulation and registration of people working in health and care. The PSA itself is overseen by Parliament. In addition to the scrutiny of professional regulators, it also

Table 4.1 Healthcare regulators overseen by the PSA in the UK.

General Chiropractic Council
General Dental Council
General Medical Council
General Optical Council
General Osteopathic Council
General Pharmaceutical Council
Health and Care Professions Council
Nursing and Midwifery Council
Pharmaceutical Society of Northern Ireland

develops standards and influences regulatory policy. The powers of the PSA are considerable and Parliament requires that reports are submitted on how well the health and social care regulators meet their responsibilities.

In addition, the organisation audits fitness to practise cases, reviewing the outcome, and can refer a regulator to the High Court (Court of Session in Scotland) if the PSA considers the outcome does not sufficiently protect the public, whether that be the finding or the sanction imposed, or both. This power is conferred under section 29 of the National Health Service Reform and Health Care Professions Act 2002. This is known as appealing a regulatory decision. When considering if an outcome is insufficient, the PSA use the following criteria. Is the outcome sufficient to:

• protect the health, safety and well-being of the public?
• maintain public confidence in the profession concerned?
• maintain proper professional standards and conduct for members of that profession?

Each of the above regulators sends decisions made by the fitness to practise committees to the PSA. If the PSA is concerned by the outcome, it can request copies of all the evidence. If the concern is unresolved then a case meeting is held to decide if a referral to court is to be made. In 2015, the PSA held six case meetings relating to GDC decisions; in 2016, five case meetings were held. In 2016, three decisions were appealed and the cases were referred to the High Court.

Regulation of Dental Services Programme Board

In September 2014, a group of organisations came together with a responsibility for setting, managing and regulating how dental care is provided in England. The group is called the Regulation of Dental Services Programme Board (RDSPB), and its formation was an initiative of the Care Quality Commission. The group aims to jointly ensure that patients receive high-quality, safe dental services from professionals and organisations that are competent and meet national standards, and that services improve.

The members of the RDSPB are:
• Care Quality Commission
• Department of Health
• General Dental Council
• NHS England.

Its work is supported and underpinned by:
• NHS Business Services Authority
• Healthwatch England and the local Healthwatch network.

The board's purpose is to review the approach to dental regulation across England and assess the effectiveness of current arrangements to develop a more streamlined, joined-up and effective model of regulation.

Health and Safety Executive

The Health and Safety Executive (HSE), the operating arm of the Health and Safety Commission, is the national independent regulator and enforcing authority for health and safety in the workplace. This covers workers in England, Scotland and Wales (including healthcare workers) and also patient and service users in Scotland and Wales. Private or publicly owned health and social care settings in Great Britain are included.

The type of issues that would be most relevant to dental practices will include:

• Reporting of Injuries, Diseases and Dangerous Occurrences Regulations 2013 (RIDDOR)
• notification of the use of ionizing radiation
• Control of Substances Hazardous to Health (COSHH).

Health and Safety Executive inspectors normally enforce health and safety standards by giving advice on how to comply with the law. Sometimes they can order individuals to make improvements by issuing them with a notice, either an Improvement Notice, which allows time for the recipient to comply, or a Prohibition Notice, which prohibits an activity until remedial action has been taken. The HSE issues notices to companies and individuals for breaches of health and safety law. The notice may involve one or more instances when the recipient has failed to comply with health and safety law; each one of these is called a 'breach'. If necessary, the HSE may prosecute recipients for non-compliance with a notice.

In 2016, five enforcement notices were given to dental workplaces. Enforcement notices are placed on the HSE website.

The HSE produces a number of helpful publications. The list below is of regulations that apply to most workplaces, including dental practices, and is taken from *Health and Safety Regulation: A Short Guide*.

1. *Management of Health and Safety at Work Regulations 1999*: requires employers to carry out risk assessments, make arrangements to implement necessary measures, appoint competent people and arrange for appropriate information and training.
2. *Workplace (Health, Safety and Welfare) Regulations 1992*: covers a wide range of basic health, safety and welfare issues such as ventilation, heating, lighting, workstations, seating and welfare facilities.
3. *Health and Safety (Display Screen Equipment) Regulations 1992*: sets out requirements for work with visual display units (VDUs).
4. *Personal Protective Equipment at Work Regulations 1992*: requires employers to provide appropriate protective clothing and equipment for their employees.
5. *Provision and Use of Work Equipment Regulations 1998*: requires that equipment provided for use at work, including machinery, is safe.

6. *Manual Handling Operations Regulations 1992*: covers the moving of objects by hand or bodily force.
7. *Health and Safety (First Aid) Regulations 1981*: covers requirements for first aid.
8. *Health and Safety Information for Employees Regulations 1989*: requires employers to display a poster telling employees what they need to know about health and safety.
9. *Employers' Liability (Compulsory Insurance) Act 1969*: requires employers to take out insurance against accidents and ill health to their employees.
10. *Reporting of Injuries, Diseases and Dangerous Occurrences Regulations 1995 (RIDDOR)*: requires employers to notify certain occupational injuries, diseases and dangerous events.
11. *Noise at Work Regulations 1989*: requires employers to take action to protect employees from hearing damage.
12. *Electricity at Work Regulations 1989*: requires people in control of electrical systems to ensure they are safe to use and maintained in a safe condition.
13. *Control of Substances Hazardous to Health Regulations 2002 (COSHH)*: requires employers to assess the risks from hazardous substances and take appropriate precautions.

Medicines and Healthcare Products Regulatory Agency

The Medicines and Healthcare Products Regulatory Agency (MHRA) regulates medicines, medical devices and blood components for transfusion in the UK. It is an executive agency, sponsored by the Department of Health.

Areas regulated by the MHRA that will be of particular relevance to dental professionals include:
- custom-made appliances
- lasers, intense light source systems and LEDs
- patient group directions
- bisphosphonates
- botulinum toxin products.

As part of its role, the MHRA has a number of activities relevant to advertising control:
- checking advertising for compliance with the law prior to publication (vetting) in clearly defined circumstances
- monitoring of published advertising material for medicines
- handling of complaints about advertising
- enforcement in relation to materials not compliant with the regulations (MHRA, 2014).

The MHRA website publishes information about companies that have been advised to amend their advertising. In the period June–August 2017, the MHRA advised 18 companies to amend their advertising of botulinum toxin products following complaints; several of the 18 were dental establishments.

Dental professionals who manufacture custom-made dental appliances are required by the Medical Devices Directive 93/42/EC to register with the MHRA, providing their business address and a description of the devices produced. This will clearly apply to dental technicians and clinical dental techniques, but will also apply to dentists who provide mouth or bite guards.

A custom-made appliance is defined by the Medical Devices Regulations 5 (1) as:

- manufactured specifically in accordance with a written prescription of a registered medical practitioner, or other person authorised to write such a prescription by virtue of his professional qualification, which gives under his responsibility, specific characteristics as to its design; and
- intended for the sole use of a particular patient.

The Human Medicines Regulations 2012 brings together most of the legislation relating to medicines in the UK, excluding the regulation of clinical trials and fees. These Regulations simplify and replace most of the Medicines Act 1968 and around 160 statutory instruments relating to medicines.

A breach of any of the provisions listed in regulation 303 is a criminal offence. This covers the vast majority of requirements set down by the Regulations. The penalty is a fine and/or imprisonment for up to 2 years in most cases. A failure to comply with any requirement imposed by a notice served under the Regulations is a criminal offence. The penalty is a fine and/or imprisonment for up to 2 years. Where the MHRA believes that a criminal offence has been committed, it will always consider enforcement action, that is, prosecution.

Right-touch regulation

As noted at the beginning of this chapter, regulation of dentistry and dental professionals is not straightforward and a number of regulators are involved. It is perhaps understandable that individuals can be confused by who does what and what regulations are applicable to dentistry.

Right-touch regulation is a description used by the PSA (2015). It outlines an approach to regulation that the PSA believes is the approach to be taken by all regulators.

'Right-touch regulation means understanding the problem before jumping to the solution. It makes sure that the level of regulation is proportionate to the level of risk to the public. It builds upon the

principles of good regulation, identified by the Better Regulation Executive, to which we added "agility". This means looking forward to anticipate change.'

The principles state that regulation should aim to be:

- *proportionate*: regulators should only intervene when necessary. Remedies should be appropriate to the risk posed, and costs identified and minimised
- *consistent*: rules and standards must be joined up and implemented fairly
- *targeted*: regulation should be focused on the problem, and minimise side effects
- *transparent*: regulators should be open, and keep regulations simple and user friendly
- *accountable*: regulators must be able to justify decisions, and be subject to public scrutiny
- *agile*: regulation must look forward and be able to adapt to anticipate change.

There are eight elements that sit at the heart of right-touch regulation.

- Identify the problem before the solution.
- Quantify and qualify the risks.
- Get as close to the problem as possible.
- Focus on the outcome.
- Use regulation only when necessary.
- Keep it simple.
- Check for unintended consequences.
- Review and respond to change.

Right-touch regulation is the minimum regulatory force required to achieve the desired result.

References

Care Quality Commission (CQC) (2010) *Guidance about Compliance: Essential Standards of Quality and Safety.* Available at: https://services.cqc.org.uk/sites/default/files/gac_-_dec_2011_update.pdf (accessed 10 January 2018).

Dental Board of the United Kingdom (1957) *Minutes with Reports of Committees, etc. for the Year 1956 and General Index to the Minutes 1921–1956.* Vol. XV.

General Dental Council (2012) *Preparing for Practice. Dental Team Learning Outcomes for Registration.* General Dental Council, London.

Health and Safety Executive (2003) *Health and Safety Regulation … A Short Guide*, Appendix 1. Available at: www.hse.gov.uk/pubns/hsc13.pdf (accessed 10 January 2018).

MHRA (2014) *Blue Guide. Advertising and Promotion of Medicines in the UK.* Available at: https://www.gov.uk/government/uploads/system/uploads/attachment_data/file/376398/Blue_Guide.pdf (accessed 11 January 2018).

Professional Standards Authority (2015) *Rethinking Regulation.* Available at: www. professionalstandards.org.uk/docs/default-source/publications/thought-paper/ rethinking-regulation-2015.pdf (accessed 10 January 2018).

Organisation websites

General Dental Council www.gdc-uk.org
General Medical Council www.gmc-uk.org
General Pharmaceutical Council www.pharmacyregulation.org
NHS England www.england.nhs.uk
Care Quality Commission www.cqc.org.uk
Healthcare Inspectorate Wales www.hiw.org.uk
NHS National Services Scotland www.nhsnss.org
NHS Scotland www.scot.nhs.uk
Practitioner Services Division www.nhsnss.org/services/practitioner
Regulation and Quality Improvement Authority www.rqia.org.uk
Health and Social Care Board www.hscboard.hscni.net
Healthwatch England www.healthwatch.co.uk
Professional Standards Authority www.professionalstandards.org.uk
Regulation of Dental Services Programme Board www.cqc.org.uk/guidance
Health and Safety Executive www.hse.gov.uk
Medicines and Healthcare Products Regulatory Agency www.gov.uk/mhra

Chapter 5   **Organisations that play a supporting role**

Should you be unfortunate enough to need them, there are a number of organisations that support dental professionals who find themselves with a complaint or concern raised about their practice. In this chapter, I will describe some of these organisations and the support they offer. The list is not exhaustive. I have subdivided the organisations into the various categories of support offered to practitioners.

- Specialist indemnity providers
- Educational support
- Health support
- Mentoring/professional support
- Advisory support

Specialist indemnity providers

Since November 2015, all dental registrants are required to have indemnity arrangements and to complete an annual declaration to the GDC that this is the case. Practising without indemnity is no longer permitted and if discovered will lead to serious consequences for the registrant.

Having indemnity is essential to ensure that patients are able to claim compensation should they need to do so without having to resort to the civil court. The patient has a right to expect this and dental professionals have a duty to ensure that right is enacted. It is an ethical as well as a statutory and regulatory duty.

There are three large specialist providers of indemnity for dentists in the UK: Dental Protection Ltd (DPL), Dental Defence Union (DDU) and Medical and Dental Defence Union of Scotland (MDDUS). All operate throughout the UK. At the time of writing, DPL and DDU provide indemnity for all registrant groups. MDDUS provides indemnity for dentists, dental hygienists, dental therapists and orthodontic therapists. Most specialist societies and associations for dental nurses, dental technicians and dental hygiene and therapy include arrangements for indemnity cover in their

How to Survive Dental Performance Difficulties, First Edition. Janine Brooks.
© 2018 John Wiley & Sons Ltd. Published 2018 by John Wiley & Sons Ltd.

membership fee. Contact your specialist society to see what arrangements it has in place.

It is a thorny problem to set the fees at a level that is acceptable to those who have not needed to use their indemnity organisation but still gives sufficient resource to support those who may require considerable help and representation. However, the knowledge that no dental professional knows when they may need the help and support of their indemnity provider makes the fees more acceptable. What we do know is that complaints against dental professionals appear to be rising, so the possibility that any one of us could need help is increasing.

All indemnity organisations offer their members/subscribers advice and support should they be the subject of a complaint. Often advice is all that is required; a telephone call can provide reassurance and assistance. However, sometimes more is needed and in cases involving fitness to practise proceedings, the indemnity organisation plays a central role in advice, guidance, support and representation of the individual. The first action for any dental professional who finds themselves the subject of a complaint, or indeed where there is the potential for a complaint, is to contact their indemnity provider.

For those dental professionals who need considerable or repeated indemnity support, there is the danger that the organisation may no longer want that individual as a member and can refuse to continue their subscription. Consequently, the dental professional must seek indemnity from a non-specialist provider. This is extremely serious, not least because once outside the 'Big 3' specialist providers, indemnity cost rise considerably and can be prohibitive. In addition, the level of professional dental advice and support available from non-specialist indemnity organisations may be minimal or non-existent. I have worked with dentists who found this out to their cost and now pay heavily for 'ordinary' insurance cover.

To minimise the possibility of your indemnity organisation refusing your continued membership, the following points are important.

- Always pay your membership fee on time – direct debits can ensure this happens.
- Ensure you have the correct category of membership.
- Pay the correct subscription rate.
- Tell your indemnity provider if your scope of practice changes.
- Ensure you complete your initial application form correctly and fully.

Educational support

Health Education England: Local Education and Training Boards

Health Education England (HEE) plans and commissions education and training for all primary care services including dentistry. Local Education and Training Boards (LETBs) are responsible for education and training at a local level and are accountable to NHS England (NHSE). They host post-graduate dental deaneries. Currently there are four LETBs in England. There are dental deaneries for Scotland, Northern Ireland and Wales.

Postgraduate dental deaneries

These provide support to dental professionals who find themselves in difficulty. They receive no specific funding to undertake the support they give. Consequently, most charge registrants for the advice given although often the first meeting is free. Support includes help to construct a personal development plan (PDP), help to build an action plan for registrants to meet the GDC determination requirements, coaching/mentoring and general advice. The deaneries provide a programme of continuing professional development (CPD) that will help those with a GDC case to complete some of the GDC requirements. For registrants with an NHS number, the courses are generally free or at low cost, although this may change as continuing efficiency savings are required of the NHS. For private practitioners, most deaneries require a fee, often one-off or an annual fee, after payment of which practitioners can attend the CPD courses.

Often meeting with the postgraduate dental dean or their representative is specifically included in a determination following either an interim orders committee hearing or a fitness to practise panel hearing. Registrants would be wise to contact their postgraduate deanery at an early stage. This will ensure there is time to undertake the work needed to complete the PDP and action plan as well as the actual remediation activities. Dental deaneries are required to commission education for all dental registrant groups, not just dentists.

Bear in mind that there have been cuts to deanery budgets and budgets for occupational health services for clinicians have also been affected. It is unlikely this situation will improve in the near future, so it is reasonable to expect to pay for the support available.

NHS Education for Scotland

NHS Education for Scotland (NES) is a special health board within NHS Scotland. It is responsible for education and training and this includes under-graduate, postgraduate and continuing professional development. NES has developed a programme (TRaMS) to support dental professionals who are struggling or for whom there is cause for concern.

Training, Revision and Mentoring Support Programme (TRaMS)

This programme offers support to all dental professionals. It includes help to develop a PDP, guidance on reflective practice, simulated clinical skills and access to a trained mentor. TRaMS can help to develop an action plan and remediation learning plan with agreed milestones. This can help to chunk up the work that is needed into manageable pieces. You will find a guidance document on the TRaMS website (TRaMS@nes.scot.nhs.uk). If an individual has a health concern or there are behavioural/attitudinal problems, TRaMS can signpost where further advice and support can be obtained. The programme also has a number of trained mentors throughout Scotland who can provide mentoring in support of remediation.

Self-referral is the most common way to access the programme, although organisations such as the health boards, indemnity organisations, Practitioner Services Division or the GDC may refer an individual. Contact can be made and a referral requested via email – see the contact details at the end of the chapter. There is a cost for the programme, so it is best to discuss that when making an enquiry. In addition, the website includes details of costs.

NHS Wales

The NHS Wales Dental Deanery works in partnership with local health boards and NHS trusts in Wales. It has a dental professional support unit which offers help with performance-related issues and remediation support. This includes support in preparing a PDP, audit and appraisal training. It also provides study days.

Northern Ireland

The Northern Ireland Medical and Dental Training Agency (NIMDTA) is responsible for providing opportunities for continuing education with courses and resources to support personal development planning for all members of the dental team. At this time, there is no specific support for those who may be struggling with a performance concern.

Committee of Postgraduate Dental Deans and Directors (COPDEND)

COPDEND is the group where all the postgraduate dental deans in England, Scotland, Northern Ireland and Wales work together. The postgraduate dental deans commission and manage the delivery of postgraduate dental education and training for the whole dental team. They also provide support for dental professionals in difficulty. COPDEND has developed a framework for support and remediation for those for whom there are performance concerns, used by all the deaneries. The support offered includes help in preparing a remediation action plan, PDP and signposting to appropriate educational activities and courses. Most deaneries also have access to trained mentors. There is a cost for the service provided.

Health support

Dentists' Health Support Trust

The Dentists' Health Support Trust (DHST) was founded in 1986 as a registered charity (www.dentistshealthsupporttrust.org). It supports a programme that provides a number of services including responding to enquiries, which may lead to intervention, assessments and treatment pathways followed by ongoing monitoring and support. The Dentists' Health Support Programme (DHSP) is a busy responsive service which gives dentists in difficulty the opportunity to make contact with highly experienced experts in the identification and management of addictive and mental health disorders. The DHSP forms an essential component of the response to the heightened illness risk experienced by dentists. Indirectly, the programme underpins good patient care by supporting dental professionals struggling with ill health and returning them to safe, valued practice in an efficient and effective way.

Support is extended to families and colleagues of the dental professional in difficulty. A vital role is that of case management where the co-ordinators take responsibility for liaison between health and other professionals involved in the dental professional's treatment/support. Support provided includes:

- advice and counselling from a mental health professional
- treatment programmes designed for each individual, to suit his/her addictive state
- inpatient treatment in an appropriate clinic for the more severely affected
- support and advice for friends, family and colleagues, who are often the first to realise that someone is ill and needs help
- assistance to return to work and support in the early years of recovery.

Practitioner Health Programme

The Practitioner Health Programme (PHP) was set up in 2008, a development originally facilitated by the NCAS (www.php.nhs.uk). It is run by the Hurley Group and provides health services to doctors and dentists living and working within the London area. It provides care and treatment to practitioners who are unable to access confidential care from mainstream NHS routes because of the nature of their role or their health condition. The programme operates in Central London and provides assessment with respect to the workplace and supports return to work. There are specialist mental health and addiction services with outpatient, inpatient and rehabilitation care. The service is free to those within the catchment area. Practitioner patients who live outside London can access the programme if their commissioner will fund the care.

As a patient of the PHP, you have the right to request that your status as a practitioner patient of the service is known only to you and the PHP.

British Doctors and Dentists Group

The British Doctors and Dentists Group (BDDG) was formed in 1973 and is a group of doctors and dentists who are recovering from, or wish to recover from, addiction, dependency on alcohol or other drugs (www.bddg.org).The group is a mutual self-help group of doctors and dentists, from all levels within the professions, who are addicted to alcohol and/or drugs and who are living, or wish to live, in a recovery programme free of alcohol and drugs.

There are 18 active BDDG groups, 17 in the UK and one in Eire, who generally meet once a month to share experiences, strengths and hopes in order to understand their common problems and to help and encourage other colleagues into recovery from their alcoholism and/or drug addiction.

Sick Doctors Trust

This group, formed in 1996, supports doctors, dentists and medical students who have drugs or alcohol addiction (www.sick-doctors-trust.co.uk). They have a helpline that offers information and advice and will also provide moral support for those who are facing regulatory hearings.

Mentoring/professional support

Local Dental Committees

Local Dental Committees (LDCs) were originally formed in 1948 at the start of the NHS. They represent the dental profession locally. They discuss issues that have local impact for dentists, for example service configuration and commissioning, NHS management of service providers, workforce planning, dental education and regulations and regulatory changes. They often provide pastoral support and other services to practitioners in the area. Practitioner advice and support schemes (PASS) are provided by many LDCs and offer important prevention and resolution aid to dentists who are struggling with their performance and may present a cause for concern. In England, LDCs often take part in NHS England's performance advisory groups (PAGs) and performers lists decision panels, which make determinations about practitioner performance. In addition, LDCs are usually involved in managed clinical networks and local dental networks, which makes them very connected and knowledgeable about national and local processes and issues.

All dentists who are on an NHS performers list are required to pay a levy to assist funding of their local LDC. Personal dental services providers and private practitioners can make voluntary contributions if they wish to be represented by their LDC. NHS community dental services and other branches of dentistry may have local agreements in place. Levies are collected on behalf of each LDC by the Business Services Authority in England and Wales, Practitioner Services in Scotland and Business Services Organisation in Northern Ireland.

An LDC can only represent those dentists who are members.There are currently 110 LDCs in England and Wales. There are also LDCs in Scotland or Northern Ireland.

Contact details for each LDC can be found on the British Dental Association website.

Dental Mentors UK

Dental Mentors UK operates an online directory of dental professionals who have experience in mentoring (and sometimes coaching) (www.dentalmentorsuk.com). It was set up by two dentists who have years of experience of mentoring for remediation. Most of the mentors in the directory have a qualification in mentoring. A number have experience in mentoring for remediation and all have considerable experience in their field of dentistry. There is information on the website about mentoring. It is free to browse the website and read the profiles and CVs of the mentors. Potential mentees pay for the mentoring they receive from the mentor of their choice.

Advisory support

National Clinical Assessment Service (NCAS)

The NCAS, originally known as the National Clinical Assessment Authority, was set up in 2001 in response to a recommendation of the 1998 Inquiry into the Bristol babies scandal (the Kennedy Inquiry) (www.ncas.nhs.uk). Initially set up for doctors, it expanded its services to dentists in 2003 and then pharmacists in 2006.

The NCAS has been an operating division of NHS Resolution (the operating name of the NHS Litigation Authority) since 2013. The NCAS provides advice and expertise to the NHS on resolving concerns fairly and sharing learning for improvement.

The NCAS aims to help the resolution of concerns about professional practice. Since 2001, over 10 000 referrals have been received from employers and contracting bodies across the UK. At any one time, the NCAS reports that it is working with around 70% of NHS organisations and each year about three in four organisations make a new referral.

NCAS services are available to NHS organisations in England, Wales and Northern Ireland.

Health boards

Wales and Scotland have a different NHS structure to England. There are regional NHS boards, 14 in Scotland and 7 in Wales. The boards are responsible for the protection and improvement of their population's health and for planning and delivery of frontline healthcare services

Practitioner Services Division

The Practitioner Services Division (PSD) works on behalf of health boards to support general practitioners, dentists, opticians, community pharmacies and dispensing contractors delivering primary care across Scotland. This includes payment, maintaining an up-to-date patient registration database, medical record transfers and clinical governance for dental services. It ensures that general dental services care and treatment are provided as required and makes payments to general dental practitioners for their services.

Conclusion

You may ask, why spend time and money supporting a dental professional who has performed poorly? Aren't there enough dental professionals to take their place? Shouldn't we just root them out of the profession, these bad apples that make everyone else look bad? I sincerely hope that if you take this view, reading this book will give you pause for thought and maybe change your thinking.

All dental professionals are expensive for society to train, dentists being the most expensive as their training takes the most time. In addition to society's contribution, each individual will pay a considerable amount for their training; they invest time, money, blood, sweat and tears. We also need to think about the time invested by those who teach and train dental professionals. Yes, I know most of them get paid to do it, but it would be soul destroying to think that your time and effort had been for nothing if the dental professional you educated was lost from the profession before their career came to a natural close. Finally, we should consider the cost to the families of those who train to be dental professionals. Make no mistake, they invest heavily as well and are likely to be devastated when their loved one struggles and faces a disciplinary or regulatory process.

So as it is very expensive to educate and train dental professionals, whenever possible the right choice is to support and help those who stumble and aid their return to safe, valued dental practice. I believe this is the ethical, humane and most cost-effective option.

References

Committee of Postgraduate Dental Deans and Directors (COPDEND) (2015) *Remediation of Dental Registrants in Difficulty. Guidance Notes on the Management of Remediation Cases Referred to Dental Postgraduate Organisations.* Committee of Postgraduate Dental Deans and Directors, Manchester.

Kennedy, I. (2002) *Learning from Bristol. The Report of the Public Inquiry into Children's Heart Surgery at the Bristol Royal Infirmary, 1984–1995.* Aailable at: http://webarchive.nationalarchives.gov.uk/20130123203804/http://www.dh.gov.uk/en/Publicationsandstatistics/Publications/PublicationsPolicyAndGuidance/DH_4002859 (accessed 10 January 2018).

Organisation websites

Specialist indemnity providers

Dental Protection Ltd www.dentalprotection.org
Dental Defence Union www.theddu.com
Medical and Dental Defence Union of Scotland www.mddus.com

Educational support

NHS Scotland, Training, Revision and Mentoring Support Programme
  TRaMS@nes.scot.nhs.uk
NHS Wales Dental Deanery walesdeanery@cardiff.ac.uk
Northern Ireland Medical and Dental Training Agency www.nimdta.gov.uk
COPDEND – for all local deanery contacts www.copdend.org

Health support

Practitioner Health Programme www.php.nhs.net
Dentists' Health Support Programme www.dentistshealthsupporttrust.org
British Doctors and Dentists Group www.bddg.org
Sick Doctors Trust www.sick-doctors-trust.co.uk

Mentoring/professional support

Local Dental Committee https://bda.org/dentists/representation/gdps/ldcs
Dental Mentors UK www.dentalmentorsuk.com

Advisory support

NCAS www.ncas.nhs.uk
Health Boards – Scotland www.gov.scot
Health Boards – Wales www.wales.nhs.uk
Practitioner Services Division www.nhsnss.org

Professional organisations

British Dental Association www.bda.org
British Association of Dental Nurses www.badn.org.uk
British Society of Dental Hygiene and Therapy www.bsdht.org.uk
Dental Technologists Association www.dta-uk.org
British Dental Industry Association www.bdia.org.uk
National Association of Dental Advisers www.nada-uk.org
British Association of Dental Therapists www.badt.org.uk
Orthodontic National Group www.orthodontic-ong.org
British Association of Clinical Dental Technology www.dentureprofessionals.
  org.uk

My apologies if I have omitted a professional organisation offering support
and advice to dental professionals.

Chapter 6 **The anatomy of a fitness to practise case**

Introduction

In 1956 when the GDC became independent of the GMC, there were 15 895 diplomates and registered graduates on the GDC register, 2827 of those registered under the provision of the 1921/23 Dental Acts (Dental Board, 1957). The new GDC developed its own professional code of ethics.

In the years before the GDC became an independent regulator (and whilst it operated under the wing of the GMC as a Dental Board; that is, 1922–1955), a total of 555 disciplinary cases were heard, an average of 16 cases each year. The number of cases ranged from eight in 1945 and 1946 to 36 in 1936. There were few clinical issues raised and the type of offences heard included embezzlement, drunkenness, living on prostitution, fornication, incest, indecent assault, canvasing and the Motor Car Act 1903. Clearly interesting times for the dental profession and of course, it was just dentists at that time. The first instance of a female dentist coming to the notice of the Dental Board was in 1932, for advertising (Dental Board, 1957).

The GDC sets the standards by which all dental professionals are measured. All dental professional groups are judged the same; the standards do not vary depending on whether you are a dentist, specialist, dental nurse, orthodontic therapist or any of the other dental professional groups that exist in the UK. The standards expected are clearly laid out in publications of the GDC; currently (2017), these can be found in *Standards for the Dental Team* (GDC, 2013).

In Chapter 2, I looked at factors that contribute to poor performance. In this chapter I will look at actual cases over a period of 3 years, 2014–2016, and the issues that were found in fitness to practise cases across all registrant groups. The aim is to show the range of issues that dental professionals struggle with and which can bring them to the attention of the regulator through complaints. Details of the cases have been extracted from the GDC annual reports and the website – the hearings and appeals section; both sources are freely available.

How to Survive Dental Performance Difficulties, First Edition. Janine Brooks.
© 2018 John Wiley & Sons Ltd. Published 2018 by John Wiley & Sons Ltd.

Before reviewing the detail of these cases, I want to set the scene and consider the number and type of dental professionals who are registered to practise dentistry in the UK (Table 6.1).

I have previously acknowledged vexatious or malicious complaints and they do occur with particularly unpleasant experiences for those who are targeted; however, I do not intend to dwell on this type of complaint. This book largely covers those complaints that are deemed to have substance. A number of complaints are found not to have substance and the case is closed at an early stage, sometimes by the case manager, sometimes by the Investigating Committee and sometimes by the Practice Committee.

Table 6.2 shows the number of each type of dental professional on the register, between 2014 and 2016. Some professionals may be qualified in more than one category, for example as a dental nurse and also as an orthodontic therapist, or as a dental technician and also as a clinical dental technician. A dental professional who has more than one title is counted once for each title that they hold. Therefore, the totals for any one year will be greater than the overall number of people. For example, in 2016, there were 1637 more titles than individuals.

Table 6.1 Total number of people on the Dentists Register and the Dental Care Professionals Register at December 2016, by gender.

Registrant group	Number of individuals	Male	Female
Dentist	41 483	21 690 (52%)	19 793 (48%)
Dental care professional	67 880	5683 (8%)	62 197 (92%)
Total	**109 363**	**27 373 (25%)**	**81 990 (75%)**

Source: GDC 2016 Annual Report.

Table 6.2 Total number of titles on the Dentists Register and Dental Care Professionals Register at the end of 2014, 2015 and 2016.

Registrant group	2014	2015	2016
Dentist	41 038 (38%)	41 095 (37%)	41 483 (37%)
Clinical dental technician	305 (<1%)	347 (<1%)	351 (<1%)
Dental hygienist	6573 (6%)	6753 (6%)	6931 (6%)
Dental nurse	52 839 (49%)	54 663 (50%)	55 525 (50%)
Dental technician	6315 (6%)	6295 (6%)	6188 (5%)
Orthodontic therapist	405 (<1%)	457 (<1%)	522 (0.5%)
Total	**107 475**	**109 610**	**111 000**

Table 6.3 Dentists: breakdown by where qualified at the end of 2014, 2015 and 2016.

Where qualified/year	2014	2015	2016
Overseas Registration Examination	2820 (7%)	2957 (7%)	3120 (8%)
Overseas qualified	1846 (5%)	1778 (4%)	1771 (4%)
UK qualified	29426 (71%)	29541 (72%)	29836 (72%)
EEA qualified	6946 (17%)	6819 (17%)	6756 (16%)
Total	**41038**	**41095**	**41483**

Sources: GDC Annual Report 2015, GDC Annual Report 2016.

The total number of registrants is increasing each year, but some registrant groups show only small increases and the number of dental technicians has decreased over the period.

The Overseas Registration Examination (ORE) is available for dentists who hold a primary dental qualification from a university that is not in either the European Economic Area (EEA) or Switzerland. Those dentists to whom this applies but who qualify as an exempt person are eligible to have their degree assessed on an individual basis. This is known as individual assessment, and unsuccessful applicants are required to sit the ORE.

Over the years 2014–2016, the proportions of registered dental professionals who are UK qualified and those who have obtained their primary qualification outside the UK have remained fairly steady (Table 6.3). In 2016, just over a quarter of registrants qualified outside the UK – 11 647 individuals.

Fitness to practise

Fitness to practise is an overarching concept which includes a number of aspects. A dental professional who is fit to practise is able to provide dental services, care and treatment safely and effectively to patients. It includes the professional's ability to undertake procedures and interventions, that is, their clinical ability and competence, skill, knowledge and expertise. It also includes behaviour and character traits demonstrated both in the practising environment and outside.

General Dental Council

'As part of our duty to protect the public, if a dentist or dental care professional falls seriously short of the standards expected of them we can either remove them from the Register or restrict what they can do professionally. These powers, given to us by Parliament, cover all

registered dentists and dental care professionals whether they are working in the NHS or in private practice.

There may be doubts about a dental professional's fitness to practise due to:

- *Health*
- *Conduct, including convictions and cautions; or*
- *Performance.*

We look carefully at every case. In some cases, we may simply offer advice rather than removing or restricting a dental professional's registration.' (www.gdc-uk.org/professionals)

The GDC reports that of the total number of registrants in a given year, only 1.8% enter the fitness to practise process, 0.3% are referred to a practice committee and 0.2% have a sanction imposed following an initial or review hearing, with 0.02% erased (GDC, 2017).

Fitness to practise process

The flowchart in Figure 6.1 is a useful summary of the fitness to practise process, what the stages are, how a registrant's case proceeds and the estimated time taken for each stage.

In 2017, the GDC fitness to practise process had four major stages and a dental registrant could expect the full process to be completed in approximately 15 months, not including appeal. The stages begin with triage or screening to determine if the issues raised in the complaint meet the 'real prospect test' which has three stages:

1. whether there is a real prospect of the facts, as alleged, being found proved (stage 1), and if so,
2. whether or not there is a real prospect of the statutory ground being established (stage 2), and if so
3. whether or not there is a real prospect of a finding of current impairment being made (stage 3) (GDC, 2016).

If it is concluded that the issues do meet the real prospect test, then the case may go to either the Interim Orders Committee or to investigation, ahead of assessment. At assessment, the case may be closed, referred to the Interim Orders Committee or go forward to case examiners. Case examiners work in pairs, one dentally qualified and one lay examiner, who are appointed as GDC staff. The outcome of this stage can include referral to the Interim Orders Committee, referral to the Investigating Committee, a warning (published or unpublished), advice to the registrant or case closed with no further action. Case examiners can also agree undertakings with the

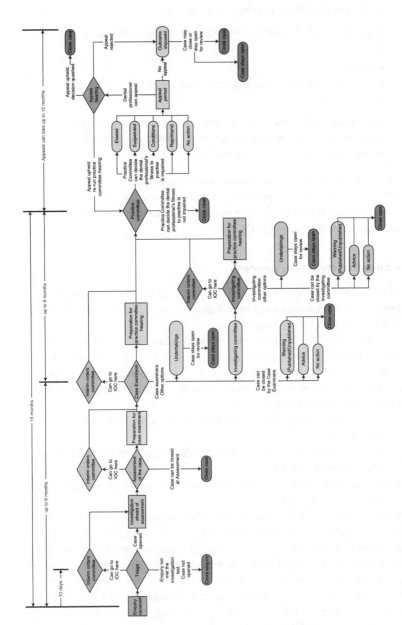

Figure 6.1 GDC fitness to practise process flowchart, showing likely duration of cases.

registrant. This means that the case is not referred on to a Practice Committee for a full hearing. In the absence of undertakings, the case can be referred to a full hearing of one of the three Practice Committees. The GDC suggests in its timeline that the time for a case to be investigated and heard by a Practice Committee should that be deemed appropriate, is currently approximately 15 months. However, if the case is not concluded at that first Practice Committee hearing and sanctions are applied then the registrant will be in the process for longer, sometimes much longer.

Case examiners were introduced in 2016 following a S60 Order. It is intended that they will take the place of the Investigating Committee as the formal decision makers and that they can conclude certain cases without the need for full fitness to practise proceedings. The Investigating Committee is not totally replaced and will still consider cases where either the registrant or the GDC solicitor challenges a Practice Committee referral. Undertakings are also newly introduced. Undertakings can be offered by case examiners only if the case would have been referred to a Practice Committee and if erasure would be an unlikely outcome.

The Interim Orders Committee remains and a case can be referred to this committee at any stage. A referral would be made because of serious patient safety issues, to protect the registrant or due to other wider public interest. In essence, this is the fast track.

Interim Orders Committee

The Interim Orders Committee (IOC) hears serious allegations quickly to decide if limits (temporary sanctions) need to be placed on a registrant's practice while their case is waiting to be heard.

> 'The role of the Interim Orders Committee is to undertake a risk assessment based on the information before it. Its role is to assess the nature and substance of any risk to the public in all the circumstances of the case and to consider whether it is necessary for the protection of the public, is otherwise in the public interest, or is in the registrant's own interests to impose an interim order on their registration. It is not the role of the IOC to make findings of facts in relation to any charge. That is the role of a differently constituted committee at a later stage in the process.'

(GDC, preface paragraph from determinations)

Investigating Committee

This committee considers allegations of impaired fitness to practise and decides if the case should be referred to a Practice Committee or the Interim Orders Committee. The committee will also consider cases where the case examiners have failed to make a determination. The objective is to consider if there is a real prospect that the allegations made against a registrant could be proved and if so, whether the registrant's fitness to practise would be impaired. This committee meets in private.

Practice Committees

There are three practice committees, which meet in public. However, where sensitive information is disclosed or discussed, there is the option for those aspects to be heard in private.

Professional Conduct Committee

The Professional Conduct Committee (PCC) considers allegations of misconduct and if proven, decides if there is an impairment of the professional's fitness to practise.

Between 2014 and 2016, the majority of fitness to practise cases were heard by the PCC.

Professional Performance Committee

The Professional Performance Committee (PPC) considers allegations of deficient performance and if proven, decides if there is an impairment of the professional's fitness to practise.

In 2014 there were seven hearings of the PPC; in 2015 there were 17 PCC hearings; in 2016, there were 26 PPC hearings, all dentists.

Health Committee

The Health Committee (HC) considers cases where it appears that either a physical or mental health condition is affecting the dental professional's fitness to practise.

In 2014, there were 21 hearings, involving 14 dentists, six dental nurses and one dental technician. In 2015, there were 33 hearings involving 25 dentists, eight dental nurses, one dental technician and one dental hygienist. In 2016, there were 15 hearings involving eight dentists, six dental nurses and one dental hygienist.

Sanctions

Fitness to practise committees are able to administer a number of sanctions. Sanctions are not supposed to be a punishment; they are imposed to protect patients and the public. However, as a dental professional, sanctions can feel to be punitive.

Warning

Issued by case examiners and may be published or not published. A warning is given when there is some evidence supporting the allegation(s) and where the registrant's conduct, practice or behaviour has fallen below the expected standard. The warning is usually for 24 months and is generally published unless the information directly relates to health, private or family life. It forms part of the registrant's fitness to practise history.

Reprimand

A reprimand is the lowest sanction that a Practice Committee can apply. It is a statement of the Committee's disapproval, but the registrant is still fit to practise with no restrictions and no other action needs to be taken. The reprimand will appear alongside the person's name on the register and forms part of their fitness to practise history. It is disclosable to employers and other registrars.

Undertakings

An undertaking is an agreement between the GDC and the registrant. It may include restriction of practice or required training. It is not used where there is a realistic chance that the registrant could be erased. It is also not appropriate where the registrant has an adverse health condition. The undertakings must be workable and are more likely to be agreed where the registrant demonstrates insight into the issues. They are generally applied for not more than 3 years and are generally published on the register for the period they apply. Compliance is monitored by the GDC case review team. Should the registrant fail or breach their undertaking then the likely result is immediate referral to a Practice Committee.

Conditions

This is where restrictions are placed on the registrant's registration for a set amount of time, up to 36 months. The conditions may include that the registrant must take further training and provide a future panel hearing with evidence to prove that they are taking steps to improve. The conditions usually have to be reviewed within a certain time. Although conditions may be tailored to fit specific circumstances, they generally follow the format set out in the Practice Committee Conditions Bank and IOC Conditions Bank, which can be found on the GDC website. Where information concerns the health of the dental professional or relates to their private and family life, it is not disclosed in the public domain and is redacted from the information on the GDC website. Conditions can be reimposed after the end of 36 months if appropriate.

Suspension

The Committee can suspend the dental professional's registration. This means that the registrant cannot work as a dental professional for a set period of time (usually up to 1 year). The minimum time that can be imposed is 3 months, but suspension can be indefinite.

Erasure

This is the most serious sanction as it removes a registrant's name from the register. This means that they can no longer work in dentistry in the UK. An individual who has been erased from the dental register can apply for restoration to the register after a minimum period of 5 years.

Should you find yourself part of the fitness to practise process, the first thing to remember is to get help, fast and early. How you respond to the first notification from the GDC has a powerful impact on the progress and outcome of your case. This can either be positive or negative. Ignoring requests or being confrontational or hostile will almost always have a negative impact. Being co-operative, sending in information on time and being respectful of the regulator will impact positively. You have to remember that the GDC has the power to take away your livelihood, so no matter whether you feel the complaint against you has substance or not, take it very, very seriously.

All hearings are formal and mostly held in public and this can seem threatening and daunting. However, generally the public is not particularly fascinated by dental fitness to practise hearings.

Determinations are published on the GDC website and are readily available for anyone who searches for a registrant by name or browses the hearings and appeals lists. This means that information about individual dental professionals is in the public domain, and patients can and do search for their dentist or any member of their practice team.

The number of complaints received by the GDC 2010–2016 is shown in Table 6.4.

Individual registrants may have more than one case in a year, so the number of complaints received will not be the same as the number of individual registrants who have been complained about.

The number of cases considered at each stage of the fitness to practise procedure can be found in Table 6.5.

In 2015, the GDC received 2786 complaints, of which 333 progressed to a hearing with a Practice Committee. Hearings involving dentists far outstrip those involving any other registrant group (Tables 6.6, 6.7, 6.8). The number of hearings is not the same as the number of individuals as one registrant may have more than one hearing in a calendar year.

Table 6.4 Number of complaints received by the GDC 2010–2016.

Year	Complaints received
2010	1401
2011	1578
2012	2278
2013	2990
2014	3099
2015	2786
2016	2630

Source: GDC Annual Reports 2014/2015/2016.

Table 6.5 Number of cases by stage of fitness to practise, 2014–2016.

Stage	2014	2015	2016
Triage	3222	2545	2550
Assessment	2567	1992	1715
Investigating Committee	1012	974	710 (647 IC, 63 CE)
Practice Committee	403	431	333 (305 IC, 28 CE)

Source: GDC Annual Reports, 2014/2015/2016.
CE, case examiner (newly introduced in 2016); IC, Investigating Committee; IOC, Interim Orders Committee.

Table 6.6 Number of IOC hearings by registrant group, 2014–2016.

	2014	2015	2016
Dentist	332	279	308
Dental nurse	56	62	66
Dental technician	35	35	24
Dental hygienist	7	7	4
Clinical dental technician	3	4	12
Therapist	1	0	0
Total hearings	**434**	**387**	**414**

Table 6.7 Interim Orders Committee outcomes, 2014–2016.

Outcome	2014	2015	2016
Interim suspension imposed	89	43	58
Interim suspension renewed	66	85	91
Interim conditions imposed	65	57	59
Interim conditions renewed	79	106	111
No order made	104	68	71
Suspension/conditions lifted	6	13	9
Adjourned	25	15	15
Total hearings	**434**	**387**	**414**

Table 6.8 PCC hearings by registrant group.

	2014	2015	2016
Dentist	160	205	220
Dental nurse	16	64	62
Dental technician	8	19	22
Dental hygienist/therapist	0	4	1
Clinical dental technician	2	2	4
Total hearings	**186**	**294**	**309**

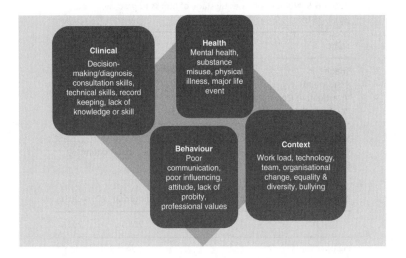

Figure 6.2 Fitness to practise issues that arise, by professional domain.

Interestingly, between 2014 and 2015 there was a four-fold rise in hearings involving dental nurses. Hearings involving dental technicians rose by 100% in 2015 compared with the year before (Figure 6.2).

Between 2014 and 2016, the number of erasures showed little variation, but the number of suspensions rose considerably. Suspensions of all types rose from 37 in 2014 to 91 in 2016 (Table 6.9).

Convictions/cautions

The number of convictions and cautions by year (all registrant groups) is shown in Table 6.10. These cases included a range of issues from assault to theft to alcohol/drugs to viewing indecent images.

Table 6.9 Outcomes for both PPC and PCC for 2014–2016 (all registrant groups). The outcomes of both committees have been added together in this table.

Outcome	2014	2015	2016
Erased with immediate suspension	33	28	31
Erased	1	0	0
Suspended with a review	23	51	86
Suspended (no review)	11	9	0
Suspended indefinitely	3	4	5
Conditions	44	54	55
Fitness to practise impaired – reprimanded	14	30	23
Fitness to practise impaired – case concluded	2	1	0
Case concluded after suspension	6	9	12
Case concluded after conditions	17	21	28
Fitness to practise not impaired	27	40	45
No misconduct	11	30	19
No case to answer	2	9	4
Total outcomes	**194**	**286**	**308**

Table 6.10 Number of convictions and cautions by year (all registrant groups).

Year	Number
2014	29
2015	41
2016	25

Note: Conviction/cautions are already counted in Practice Committee hearings – therefore not counted in the overall totals.

Analysis

The GDC publishes requirements that all dental professionals must demonstrate at the end of their training in order to be eligible to enter the register. The requirements or outcomes can be found in *Preparing for Practice* (GDC, 2015). They are divided into four domains, all of which must be attained: clinical; professional; communication; management and leadership. Figures 6.3–6.5 show the issues raised in determinations following Practice Committee hearings in 2014–2016, grouped by domain. These three figures demonstrate the breadth of issues found during fitness to practise hearings in the three years 2014–2016.

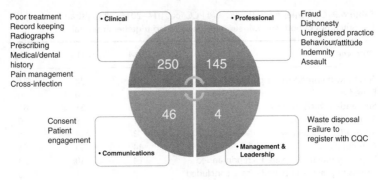

Figure 6.3 Cases by issues found 2014, analysed by GDC *Preparing for Practice* domains.

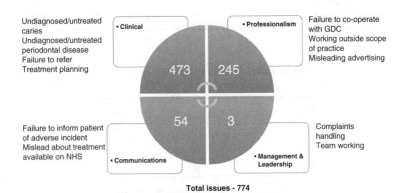

Figure 6.4 Cases by issues found 2015, analysed by GDC *Preparing for Practice* domains.

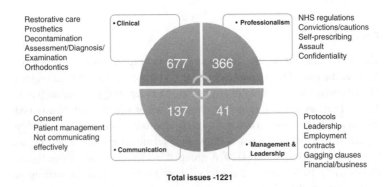

Figure 6.5 Cases by issues found 2016, analysed by GDC *Preparing for Practice* domains.

Table 6.11 Issues found against registrants by GDC domain, 2014–2016.

Issues by domain	2014	2015	2016
Clinical	250 (56%)	473 (61%)	677 (56%)
Professional	145 (33%)	245 (32%)	366 (30%)
Communication	46 (10%)	54 (7%)	137 (11%)
Management and leadership	4 (1%)	3 (>1%)	41 (3%)
Total	**445**	**775**	**1221**

The issues found against registrants by GDC domain, 2014–2016, are detailed in Table 6.11. The majority of cases will have a number of findings, so the number of issues found are in excess of the number of hearings held. This table brings together the findings in the three figures to show the number of issues raised against registrants across all registrant groups in the period 2014–2016. For each year, the greatest proportion of issues was within the clinical domain. It is of interest that the actual number of issues found against registrants has risen considerably over the period, from 445 in 2014 to 1221 in 2016.

Most common findings
The findings are similar across the period, with the most common in each year being the same: record keeping, radiographs and consent. Dishonesty is close behind along with prescribing and treatment planning. Of the clinical concerns, caries and periodontal disease (recognition and treatment) are found in many cases.

There is a strong message to be found in this analysis. The most frequent issues found in cases heard by the Practice Committees are regular, basic dental issues, perhaps with the exception of honesty and communication. It seems that some dental professionals are failing to provide the basic tenets of patient care and treatment. The more important message is that these are topics that should figure in all dental professionals' continuing professional development.

It is interesting to note that although the total number of complaints received by the GDC in 2016 was less than in 2015 (a fall of 156), this did not translate to a fall in cases heard by Practice Committees, which rose in 2016 by 17. The numbers are small when compared with the total number of registrants, but it remains to be seen whether this is a trend or a blip. **Note:** Some health cases do not disclose the hearing outcomes to the public domain.

The majority of determinations in 2015 placed conditions on the registrants' practice (37%). This was also the case in 2016, with conditions placed on 41 registrants (34%). Both these years are an increase on 2014 when 23% of cases heard had conditions placed on the registrant.

Erasure

This must surely be the worst nightmare of all dental professionals. All the years of hard work to get into training in the first place, then all the hard work to become qualified, and finally all the years given to the profession and service to patients – gone. Erasure means that the individual is removed from the dental register; they are no longer a dental professional and can no longer work in dentistry. Their dental career is over. It is possible to apply for restoration to the register, but this cannot be considered until 5 years have elapsed and the number of cases restored are small.

Between 2010 and the end of 2016, there were 10 restoration applications received from dentists erased from the register. Four were successful and in each of these cases, the dentist was restored with conditions placed upon their registration (personal communication).

The GDC states:

> 'Erasure will be appropriate when the behaviour is fundamentally incompatible with being a dental professional: any of the following factors, or a combination of them, may point to such a conclusion:
> - serious departure(s) from the relevant professional standards;
> - where a continuing risk of serious harm to patients or other persons is identified;
> - serious dishonesty, particularly where persistent or covered up;
> - a persistent lack of insight into the seriousness of actions or their consequences.'

(GDC determination, case heard on 21.1.16)

Table 6.12 shows an analysis of erasure outcomes, by registrant group and underpinning factors, for 2015. In 2015 there were no erasures for clinical dental technicians, dental therapists or dental hygienists.

Of the 319 hearings, 29 registrants were erased by the GDC. However, the proportion of cases that concluded in erasure is not evenly spread across registrant groups. Whilst only 19 dental nurses were involved in fitness to practise hearings, about half of those resulted in erasure. Fifty three of the cases across all registrant groups heard during 2015 noted a finding of dishonesty; 29 of those cases concluded with the erasure of the registrant (over half).

Table 6.13 shows an analysis of erasure outcomes, by registrant group and underpinning factors, for 2016. In 2016 there were no erasures for clinical dental technicians, dental therapists or dental hygienists.

Table 6.12 Analysis of erasure outcomes, by registrant group and underpinning factors, 2015.

Group	Number	Underpinning factors
Dentist	17	1. Sexual assault
		2. Failure to maintain appropriate indemnity, misleading, dishonest
		3. Inappropriate behaviour, sexually motivated
		4. Clinical treatment, record keeping, diagnosis and treatment planning, radiographs, antibiotic prescribing, dishonest claims
		5. Conviction 8 charges, recording a person doing a private act contrary to Sexual Offences Act 2003 – voyeurism
		6. Retired from practice April 2016. No indemnity, dishonest, clinical failures, private care when not registered with RQIA
		7. Serious failings – assessments and treatment, record keeping, failure to diagnose periodontal disease, use of radiographs
		8. Poor standard of restorative treatment, use of radiographs, periodontal assessment recording, consent, antibiotic prescribing. Dishonesty – 'doctored' notes. Fraudulent
		9. Unprofessional, misleading, financially motivated, dishonest, record keeping, informed consent. Sarcastic and rude
		10. Appeal against decision to erase – non-compliance with CPD for 2008–2013 cycle
		11. Misleading. Dishonest, inaccurate information supplied for registration with GDC
		12. Breach of patient consent. Poor standard of care provided; failing to assess and treat pain; failing to assess periodontal condition; failing to gain informed consent on more than one occasion, clinical failings fell far below the standards expected of a registered dental professional. Record-keeping failures over a protracted period of time were of a sufficiently low standard that it would be considered deplorable by fellow practitioners
		13. Did not carry out or record any or any adequate general dental examination and orthodontic clinical examination. Inadequate recording of a radiographic report. All options for treatment including no treatment discussed. All the risks of the proposed treatment discussed. Communicating with the patient's general dental practitioner (GDP). Informed consent for change in type of aligners. Full and accurate information about reasons for delay in treatment. Multiple findings of misleading and dishonest conduct. This type of misconduct which involves dishonesty and attitudinal concerns is not easily remediable
		14. False entries in records. Reckless prescribing. Dishonesty. Serious deep-seated professional attitudinal problems and behaved in a way which is fundamentally incompatible with continued registration

(Continued overleaf)

Table 6.12 (Continued)

Group	Number	Underpinning factors
		15. Provided dental services whilst not registered with the GDC (2 yrs). No indemnity (5 yrs). Undisclosed health condition. Standard of care inadequate. Record keeping unsatisfactory
		16. Clinical failures and record-keeping failures, as well as dishonest conduct in making inappropriate claims. Attitudinal issues
		17. Failed to pay ARF. Breach of honesty and integrity. Refused to co-operate with regulatory body
		Of the 17 dentists who were erased from the register in 2015, only two were erased solely for clinical failings. Non-clinical failings of behaviour, attitude or professionalism were found either alone or in combination with clinical issues in the majority of cases. Dishonesty figured in 10 cases. Dishonesty in any case is a very serious finding and is the most common behavioural trait that the GDC feels is incompatible with continuing as a dental professional.
Dental nurse	10	1. Fraud, dishonesty, integrity
		2. Assault (6/12 imprisonment)
		3. Theft conviction
		4. Misleading, dishonest
		5. Theft from employer. Failed to disclose to GDC. Dishonesty
		6. Stole cash from practice. Did not inform GDC of conviction. Dishonest
		7. Caution from police. Possession of cocaine, did not disclose to GDC. Signed self-declaration, ticked no. Conviction for wrongful credit. Misleading, dishonest
		8. Misconduct, conviction theft from employer
		9. Dishonesty, misleading. Fraudulent copy of DBS certificate. Failure to inform employer of GDC interim suspension order. Told GDC no convictions
		10. Dishonesty. Unprofessional. Providing immigration and employment services when not authorised to do so
		All 10 dental nurse registrants who were erased from the register in 2015 were found to demonstrate behaviour/attitude/professional issues. In addition, nine of the 10 registrants were found to show failings of honesty. Five of the 10 cases included theft from their employer.
Dental technician	2	1. Convicted of illegally practising dentistry. Dishonest
		2. Outside scope of practice. Claimed to be CDT. Making dentures in the absence of a prescription from a dentist. Dishonest, false claims about qualifications
		Two dental technician registrants were erased from the register in 2015; both cases were found to demonstrate dishonesty and both included working outside their scope of practice.
Total	**29**	

Table 6.13 Analysis of erasure outcomes, by registrant group and underpinning factors, 2016.

Group	Number	Underpinning factors
Dentist	20	1. Lack of indemnity, misleading, dishonest, serious attitudinal problems
		2. Infection control, reuse of single-use items, dishonesty
		3. Physical assault on a patient, left an outpatient clinic early without reasonable explanation. Dishonest representation of the GDC
		4. Assessment and diagnosis, caries diagnosis and treatment, prescribing, cross-infection, no gloves, periodontal monitoring, endodontics, radiographs, record keeping. Attitudinal issues
		5. Criminal convictions; working as a dentist whilst unregistered. Had not paid ARF, dishonest completion of re-registration form
		6. Lack of indemnity, dishonest, radiographs, treatment planning, preventive care, record keeping, endodontics, restorative care
		7. Assessment, treatment planning, consent, poor treatment, behaviour towards a colleague, implants, radiography, cross-infection, record keeping
		8. Conviction, imprisonment, fraudulent claims
		9. Clinical failings, dishonesty, radiography, consent, prescribing
		10. Forged indemnity, dishonesty
		11. Dishonesty, assessment and diagnosis, treatment planning, consent, record keeping, professional boundaries 'hugging, kissing+sex', indemnity, confidentiality
		12. Conviction, false accounting, fraud against NHS
		13. Splitting courses of treatment, dishonesty, providing private treatment to NHS patients
		14. Assessment, diagnoses, consent, standard of treatment, record keeping, crown and bridge, cross-infection, protocols, failure to co-operate with GDC
		15. Cross-infection, decontamination, failure to ensure nurse used appropriate cross-infection and decontamination, prescribing, inadequate assessment
		16. Medical history, treatment planning, consent, assessments and charting, diagnosis and treatment of caries and periodontal disease, need for specialist referral, record keeping, radiography, prescribing, provision of relevant advice

(Continued overleaf)

Table 6.13 (Continued)

Group	Number	Underpinning factors
		17. Indemnity, dishonesty – lying to GDC
		18. Radiography, periodontal disease, adequate examination and assessment, endodontics, prescribing, record keeping, consent
		19. Consent, treatment planning, communications, record keeping, radiography, failed to co-operate with GDC, indemnity, dishonesty
		20. Conviction – assault and rape. Threats to kill
		Of the 20 dentists who were erased from the register in 2016, only three were erased solely for clinical failings. Non-clinical failings of behaviour, attitude or professionalism was found either alone or in combination with clinical issues in the majority of cases. Dishonesty figured in 13 cases. Dishonesty in any case is a very serious finding and is the most common behavioural trait that the GDC feels is incompatible with continuing as a dental professional.
Dental nurse	9	1. Prescription fraud, dishonesty. Police caution
		2. Infection control, dishonestly responded to an investigation
		3. Outside scope of practice. Tooth whitening, dishonesty
		4. Theft, dishonesty
		5. Caution for burglary, failure to inform GDC, dishonesty
		6. Outside scope of practice, surgical procedure
		7. Dishonesty which was premeditated and included an attempt to cover up, misconduct which was sustained over a period of time, a blatant disregard for role as a registered professional and the role of the GDC as regulator
		8. Out of scope, misleading advertising, indemnity, dishonesty
		9. Dishonest – repeated, lied about training
		All nine dental nurse registrants who were erased from the register in 2016 were found to demonstrate behaviour/attitude/professional issues. In addition, all were found to show failings of honesty. Three of the nine cases included theft from their employer.
Dental technician	3	1. Out of scope, dishonesty
		2. Dishonesty, scope of practice, no indemnity
		3. Out of scope, dishonest, stated CDT – not qualified, inappropriate advertising
		Three dental technician registrants were erased from the register in 2016; all cases were found to demonstrate dishonesty and two included working outside their scope of practice.
Total	32	

Table 6.14 Erasures 2010 – 2016 (all registrant groups).

	2010	2011	2012	2013	2014	2015	2016
Erased/erased with immediate suspension	22	25	25	15	28	29	32

Of the 323 hearings, 32 registrants were erased by the GDC. However, the proportion of cases that concluded in erasure is not evenly spread across registrant groups. Whilst 62 dental nurses were involved in fitness to practise hearings, nine of those resulted in erasure. Overall, of cases heard by all Practice Committees in 2016, 8% of hearings of dentists, 13% of hearings of dental nurses and 14% of hearings of dental technicians ended in erasure.

Thirty five of the cases across all registrant groups heard during 2016 noted a finding of dishonesty; 25 of those cases concluded with the erasure of the registrant (just below three-quarters).

From these figures and those for 2015, it is fair to conclude that dishonesty, if found, results in a serious outcome for the registrant.

Table 6.14 shows erasures for all registrant groups, 2010–2016. While the numbers of registrants erased in both 2015 and 2016 are low, it appears that the likelihood of erasure is greater for non-dentist registrants.

Conclusion

Where a case is found to have substance, it is important that the professional shows insight and recognises that errors or mistakes have occurred and there is learning to be uncovered. If that attitude is taken then it is far more likely that the panel will take a measured approach with their determination. Dental professionals who refuse to acknowledge that their practice can improve or, worse, that there is no issue and the problem lies with a corrupt regulator or an ungrateful patient are far more likely to find their practice limited, occasionally seriously. It can be hard to find the silver lining in a complaint but if you can, it can be a turning point. I have worked with dental professionals who told me that their GDC case acted as a 'wake-up' call and helped them get back to being the practitioner they wanted to be.

When reading GDC determinations, the term 'insight' turns up quite frequently. If a professional is deemed by the panel to demonstrate insight, then the panel feel more reassured that the poor performance is less likely to be repeated. Insight includes the ability to self-analyse and reflect on the underpinning and contributory factors that produce our actions. If we have insight we are much more likely to learn from experiences, both good and not so good. A professional who is deemed not to demonstrate insight does not reassure the hearing panel that any learning has taken place, so the poor performance could be repeated. In this case, conditions are much more likely to be imposed, perhaps even a harsher outcome such as suspension or erasure. Insight and self-awareness are covered in more detail in Chapter 8.

References

Dental Board of the United Kingdom (1957) *Minutes with Reports of Committees, etc. for the Year 1956 and General Index to the Minutes 1921–1956.* Vol. XV.

General Dental Council (GDC) (2013) *Standards for the Dental Team.* General Dental Council, London.

General Dental Council (GDC) (2015) *Preparing for Practice.* General Dental Council, London.

General Dental Council (GDC) (2016) *Case Examiners Guidance Manual.* General Dental Council, London.

General Dental Council (GDC) (2017) *Guidance for Decision-Makers on the Impact of Criminal Convictions and Cautions.* General Dental Council, London.

Chapter 7 The registrant's journey, personal statements and case studies

'There are only two or three human stories, and they go on repeating themselves as fiercely as if they had never happened before.'

(Willa Cather, 1913)

This chapter contains a number of personal statements from registrants I have been privileged to work with who have personal experience of fitness to practise. I am indebted to them for sharing their stories so generously. I have also included some anonymised case studies as summaries of particular difficulties that dental professionals struggle with and their impact on performance.

The regulatory system in the UK enables anyone to raise a complaint against a dental professional. The complaint does not need to have substance or, indeed, to be true or even accurate, the object being that all complaints are dealt with seriously until proven to be otherwise. It is not necessary to put your name to the complaint you raise or identify yourself in any way.

There may be understandable reasons for allowing anonymity, particularly where a patient does not wish to be known to the professional they have a grievance against. However, this does raise the spectre of malicious or vexatious complaints. In addition, it is impossible for the GDC to properly investigate a specific complaint for a patient who wishes to remain anonymous. An anonymous complaint will still be investigated by the GDC and the dental professional involved will still go through the process, but they will be in the dark about who is dissatisfied with them. From the professional's point of view, this adds another dimension of worry and concern – if you don't know who is unhappy with you, you begin to speculate. An anonymous complaint is particularly likely to raise anxiety levels for the professional concerned.

Complaints are not only raised by patients. Dental professionals can make complaints about other dental professionals. Such complaints can also be anonymous, presumably because the person raising the complaint knows

How to Survive Dental Performance Difficulties, First Edition. Janine Brooks.
© 2018 John Wiley & Sons Ltd. Published 2018 by John Wiley & Sons Ltd.

the individual they wish to complain about. Again, this may be understandable where one dental professional employs another, as in the case of a dental nurse wishing to raise a legitimate concern about the dentist employing them. Or in the case of an associate wishing to raise a concern about their practice principal. However, the question must be why the individual making the complaint felt unable to discuss the issue with their colleague and attempt to resolve the problem locally. Of course, this may well have happened and had no effect, or the issue could seriously affect patient safety. However, a number are likely to be the result of personal animosity and the breakdown of professional relationships. The GDC appears to be ill equipped to deal with this category of complaint.

It is well understood that all dental professionals have a duty to refer colleagues who are placing patient safety at risk. If they do not, then their own registration is at risk. All dental registrants share a joint responsibility to maintain professional standards. Carrying out that responsibility is not a simple nor an easily undertaken duty, particularly if you are a younger, less experienced or junior member of the profession. The GDC (2016) has recognised that difficulty and published guidance to help.

How it can begin

Unless you have been the subject of a complaint to the GDC, it's hard to imagine what it's like. The first you will know about it is a letter from a case manager outlining that a complaint has been received, brief details of the complaint and whether it is anonymous or not. You will also be asked to complete an information template giving details about your contracts and employment status. Finally, there will be a request for a copy of your current indemnity certificate. This is the first day when your anxiety levels begin to rise. It's truly a heart sinking moment and most people react initially in a number of ways.

- Disbelief – this must be a mistake
- Anger – why has this happened?
- Denial – this is not happening
- Crushed – I must be a bad person

Very often, all four reactions will occur, sometimes together, sometimes sequentially. The emotions ebb and flow.

Your first action should be to contact your indemnity provider to alert them to the complaint and to take their advice. Very often, the letter won't have been opened until you return from work, so it will be after routine working hours. If you are really unlucky it will be a Friday evening.

Next, complete the paperwork requested as fully as possible, take copies and send them to your indemnity adviser.

This is a very trying and anxious time regardless of whether you believe the complaint to have substance or not.

Do not expect your case to be concluded quickly; it can be months or years before conclusion. Postponements happen and cases can be adjourned if the panel wishes to request more information. Be prepared for the highs and lows this can produce.

Some dental professionals decide to represent themselves at a panel hearing. My advice would be to think very, very seriously before representing yourself. The indemnity organisations, their advisers and legal professionals are skilled and experienced in GDC cases and processes, they know how to present cases and how to interpret the issues involved. They know how to guide you in preparing evidence and yourself for hearings. They can help you present yourself in the best manner possible.

If at all possible, I recommend you work with a personal mentor or coach. You should expect to pay for this; a number of dental professionals have taken further qualifications in mentoring and/or coaching and will be able to support you. I cannot emphasise enough how important it can be to have an independent professional working with you. An experienced mentor provides professional help with personal development plans, audit and reflective learning and they will usually provide a report that you can include in your evidence to the panel hearing. Along with this invaluable professional support, the personal support of having a fellow dental professional to talk to cannot be overestimated. A coach or mentor will not do the work for you nor can they guarantee your case will progress smoothly but they can signpost and guide you in the right direction.

The Hero's Journey

Before the case studies, I want to introduce you to a piece of work that I became aware of when I was completing my coach training. It resonated with me in a number of ways. I'm going to describe the work first and then explain why I think it's important to this chapter.

Joseph Campbell (1904 –1987), an American mythologist, first described what he called a pattern of narrative in hero myths and storytelling. He compared mythical stories from across the world and found an empirical thread or story in them all. He felt the basic pattern to be global and present in all human societies and cultures across the world and stretching back in time. He called the basic story the Hero's Journey (Campbell, 2014). You can find the outline he describes in almost every story you will read or film you will see. The work of Campbell inspired George Lucas (*Star Wars*) and Richard Adams (*Watership Down*), to highlight just two iconic films.

Outline of the Hero's Journey

There are 12 stages to the Hero's Journey and I will introduce them using the original language of Christopher Vogler in his work *The Writer's Journey* (1992). Later, I will elaborate on why I feel this model is an important way of looking at the 'journey' of dental professionals who find themselves facing GDC procedures.

Stages of the Hero's Journey

1. **The Ordinary World**. The hero, uneasy, uncomfortable or unaware, is introduced sympathetically so the audience can identify with the situation or dilemma. The hero is shown against a background of environment, heredity and personal history. Some kind of polarity in the hero's life is pulling in different directions and causing stress.
2. **The Call to Adventure**. Something shakes up the situation, either from external pressures or from something rising up from deep within, so the hero must face the beginnings of change.
3. **Refusal of the Call**. The hero feels the fear of the unknown and tries to turn away from the adventure, however briefly.
4. **Meeting with the Mentor**. The hero comes across a seasoned traveller of the world who gives him or her training, equipment or advice that will help on the journey. Or the hero reaches within to a source of courage and wisdom.
5. **Crossing the Threshold**. The hero commits to leaving the Ordinary World and entering a new region or condition with unfamiliar rules and values.
6. **Tests, Allies and Enemies**. The hero is tested and sorts out allegiances in the Special World.
7. **Approach**. The hero and newfound allies prepare for the major challenge in the Special World.
8. **The Ordeal**. Near the middle of the story, the hero enters a central space in the Special World and confronts death or faces his or her greatest fear.
9. **The Reward**. The hero takes possession of the treasure won by facing the ordeal. There may be celebration, but there is also danger of losing the treasure again.
10. **The Road Back**. About three-fourths of the way through the story, the hero is driven to complete the adventure, leaving the Special World to be sure the treasure is brought home.
11. **The Resurrection**. At the climax, the hero is severely tested once more on the threshold of home. He or she is purified by a last sacrifice, another moment of death and rebirth, but on a higher and more complete level. By the hero's action, the polarities that were in conflict at the beginning are finally resolved.

12. **Return with the Elixir**. The hero returns home or continues the journey, bearing some element of the treasure that has the power to transform the world as the hero has been transformed.

These stages are shown in Figure 7.1 as the hero passes from their Ordinary World into the Special World and then back again.

So, let me introduce the Registrant's Journey using the model in Figure 7.1 as the basis.

You may be wondering why I have shared with you the essential plot of most films, books and stories that you have ever read. I'm sure those of you who enjoy science fiction will have noticed the storyboards of *Star Wars* or *Galaxy Quest*, others the outline of James Bond stories or others the *Wizard of Oz*. Let's not forget Neo in *The Matrix* or Frodo in *The Lord of the Rings*.

When I first began thinking about this model it struck me how it could be applied to the stages dental professionals go through when faced with a performance issue, particularly one in which the GDC is involved. In the stages of the hero's inner journey shown in Figure 7.1, I found a resonance for the path many of those I coach or mentor pass through. Please do not misconstrue my meaning – I am not suggesting that those for whom there are performance

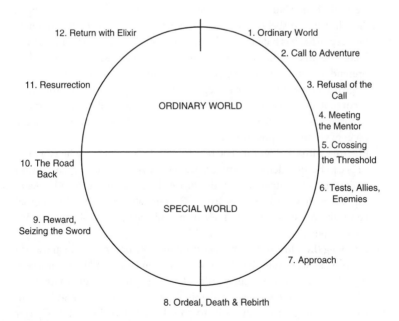

Figure 7.1 The Hero's Journey.

concerns are traditional heroes or heroines in the strict sense of the words – it is the stages of the journey that spoke to me, rather than the title.

You may feel that some of the words used to describe the stages are a little extreme or sensational. Try not to let that get in the way of the meaning. I'm going to take the stages of the Hero's (Registrant's) Journey and translate them into how they could describe the fitness to practise process for a dental professional.

1. **The Ordinary World.** The registrant is a dental professional, just like most of the professionals on the GDC register. The rest of the profession, particularly their specific professional group, dentist, nurse, technician, hygienist, can identify with them; they have all gone through rigorous education, all worked in similar environments offering the same interventions for patients. They are undertaking their regular, routine day-to-day work unaware of problems or issues that may exist.

2. **The Call to Change.** Something shakes up the regular routine, either from external pressures or something from deep within the person, so the registrant must face the beginnings of change. This stage could be represented by a complaint being received, a letter from the GDC. In the traditional model, 'Call to Adventure' is the title for this stage. I have preferred to alter the title to 'Call to Change' as I feel 'Call to Adventure' chimes less with performance concerns.

3. **Refusal of the Call.** The registrant feels a mixture of emotions – anger, denial, shame, disbelief. Often fear is experienced, often an unwillingness to accept what has happened. The urge to ignore the letter or conversation is considerable, perhaps overwhelming. There can be the response of 'let's pretend the letter was never delivered'. Some registrants stay in this stage for a long time, some rail against the process, convinced the GDC is corrupt, there is a conspiracy, denying there is a problem and everyone else is at fault. A very few never move from this stage; in those cases the outcome is rarely a positive one.

4. **Meeting with the Mentor.** The registrant talks to someone who can help. This can be an indemnity adviser, deanery adviser, mentor or coach who understands the fitness to practise proceedings and gives them help and support as they prepare for hearings. Occasionally, this can be an internal voice, the registrant finding their own resilience and resolving to move forward positively.

5. **Crossing the Threshold.** The registrant moves from their ordinary world of everyday work into the special world of regulation and GDC proceedings. There are most definitely unfamiliar rules, processes and values here. This can seem a dark place, inhabited by aliens who speak a different language. Going back to the ordinary world is not an option; fear and anger are common emotions experienced by those who cross the threshold.

6. **Tests, Allies and Enemies**. The registrant finds out who can really help and support them and who is less than helpful, occasionally even obstructive. Sometimes colleagues that the registrant had thought would support them turn away, resulting in feelings of betrayal. The registrant learns about lawyers, barristers, GDC case workers, colleagues and advisers. The costs of the process begin to dawn on the registrant. Costs are far more than just financial and will include the health of the registrant as the weight of the process begins to bear down upon them.

7. **Approach**. The registrant begins to prepare for the initial hearing, possibly an investigating committee, possibly a clinical examiner. This may include the registrant in undertaking audits, reflective writing and a personal development plan. Those who work with a coach or mentor may find it easier to prepare during the approach. Those who still bear hostile feelings may still be in 'fight' mode.

8. **The Ordeal**. The registrant attends a fitness to practise committee panel hearing. This is a very nerve-racking and anxious time. It is one of the greatest ordeals a professional can face. There is fear about the outcome and the future. The ordeal can last many months and even years. It is often composed of a number of ordeals, each hearing being an ordeal in itself, contributing to the overall process. The result of the ordeal is largely divided into two outcomes: the registrant remains in dentistry or the registrant is erased from the register. Whatever the outcome, a new life begins.

9. **The Reward**. The registrant may remain in the profession (the reward), even if conditions are placed upon practice. For those who are erased and must begin a new life outside dentistry, the reward may be a new career. Sometimes it can be difficult to recognise this stage at the time it is entered. For those who have had conditions set on their practice, there remains anxiety about satisfactory achievement of the conditions. This is the danger of losing the treasure (continued registration) again. This can be a very trying place to be and many registrants' health can suffer. Resilience and stamina can be tested to the extreme and support is crucial.

10. **The Road Back**. The registrant must work to complete the conditions on their practice. This generally means working with others, for example colleagues in the practice, indemnity adviser, deanery adviser, mentor, coach, solicitor. It can be hard working with a supervisor and feeling judged. Some registrants must find a new place to work as their old employer/practice no longer wishes to have them. The registrant is on the road back, but there are still hurdles to jump. Sometimes there is the worry that the GDC fitness to practise panel may decide insufficient progress has been made and impose further sanctions. There can still be dragons on the road back.

11. **The Resurrection**. I see this stage as being the final fitness to practise hearing where it is determined if all conditions have been satisfactorily met and from which the registrant can move on, the process behind them. The registrant has been changed; those who have reflected well on the process and the actions that lead to the referral are stronger and fitter. The tests are severe, but they have survived and even thrived; they are a better registrant (if the lessons learnt are truly embedded).

12. **Return with the Elixir**. The registrant returns to work and their life, the GDC process closed. Those who truly survive and thrive have changed their practice, their behaviour, their attitude, etc. They have learnt from the experience, improved their practice and are better professionals. This knowledge can transform their working life and others can benefit, be that colleagues or patients.

The stages are represented like a journey that is travelled in a linear fashion. This is not always the case and often the stages loop, particularly with stages 6–9. This loop can be seen where a number of panel hearings take place over a period of time, the registrant preparing evidence for the panel to deliberate. Sometimes hearings are postponed, so the ordeal is protracted. Often conditions are placed on the registrant for a number of months or years with interim reviews, each being seen as a loop.

I have used the model to represent the stages that registrants generally go through as they progress through fitness to practise proceedings. Of course, I'm sure you can see how the model could apply to many changes throughout our careers and indeed our lives.

The work of Campbell went further to look at the Hero's Inner Journey. Here, the resonance with a dental professional facing a fitness to practise hearing is more obvious (Figure 7.2).

1. Limited awareness of problem
2. Increased awareness of need to change
3. Fear, resistance to change
4. Overcoming fear
5. Committing to change
6. Experimenting with new conditions
7. Preparing for major change
8. Big change
9. Accepting consequences of new life
10. New challenge and rededication
11. Last-minute dangers
12. Mastery

This model can illuminate where on the journey a registrant is and what the remaining journey may hold. The original work may create a 'light bulb' moment for some.

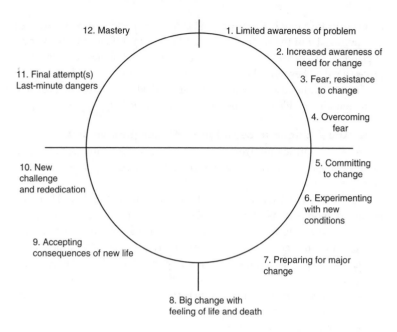

12. Mastery

1. Limited awareness of problem

2. Increased awareness of need for change

11. Final attempt(s) Last-minute dangers

3. Fear, resistance to change

4. Overcoming fear

10. New challenge and rededication

5. Committing to change

6. Experimenting with new conditions

9. Accepting consequences of new life

7. Preparing for major change

8. Big change with feeling of life and death

Figure 7.2 The Hero's Inner Journey.

Case studies

Unless you are a professional and a registrant, it can be hard to appreciate just how devastating it is to receive a fitness to practise letter from the GDC. Even a few dental professionals fail to understand the significance initially. The vast majority of dental professionals want to do a good job for every patient. We are in service to our patients, we place their interests first, we are professionals, our work is integral to our being and it often defines us. Calling into question our fitness to practise cuts to the core of who we are. The GDC has the ability to take away our registration, our livelihood. This means a dramatic effect on our self-image and our lifestyle. The prospect is a frightening one. If you cease to be a dental professional, who are you? This goes some way to explaining why a GDC investigation is such a stressful experience. Chapter 10 includes a section on neurological levels and this can help to shed light on why dental professionals become so stressed by a concern being raised about their performance.

I believe one of the best ways to understand a GDC referral is to hear from those who have experienced it first hand. I am indebted to the following colleagues who generously agreed to share their stories in the spirit of helping others who are either in the process of having their performance investigated or who may be in the future. This must have been difficult for them and I applaud the resilience they demonstrate and their willingness to help fellow professionals. They have chosen to remain anonymous.

The case studies use the words of the individuals who have kindly shared them, but I have added in my own observations in italics.

Case study 1: general dental practitioner (known as XX)

XX received notification from the GDC about a complaint against them in May 2009; the case was finally concluded in June 2014, just over 5 years later.

Referrals to the GDC are generally not concluded quickly. There are obviously good reasons why a referral takes some time to be robustly investigated and the GDC has made progress in reducing the time registrants are in the fitness to practise system. However, progress can be protracted and this factor can lead to serious anxiety, worry and ill health for the registrant concerned.

The allegations made against XX included:
- breaches in cross-infection control
- breach in practice management
- clinical issues: antimicrobial prescribing; radiograph quality assurance; caries; periodontal assessment and treatment
- motivated by financial self-interest, by allowing UDA targets to adversely affect the quality of care provided.

It is my experience from years of supporting practitioners with fitness to practise cases that the majority of cases involve relatively basic dentistry.

A total of 21 conditions were applied to XX's GDC registration for 3 years, and included carrying out six clinical audits, PDP reviewed by the deanery, having a mentor, workplace supervisor and a professional colleague, and never to work in single-handed practice.

All the conditions were removed in June 2014.

Conditions imposed on a registrant's practice are generally derived from a conditions bank that fitness to practse panels access when deciding which conditions are appropriate for a specific case. This has the advantage of enhancing consistency. Undertaking audit, reflective learning, a PDP, working with the deanery, mentors, workplace supervisors and reporters are common conditions and would be applied to a majority of cases.

I asked XX how they felt during the process.

'I felt continually stressed and under pressure, and in the spotlight. I couldn't breath and felt suffocated especially when I was cross-examined in the hearing itself. Too many thoughts were entering my mind, especially in the hearing, and I couldn't even put sentences together, to give a robust defence for the panel. I felt like a 'cat on a hot tin roof' when I returned back to clinical "hands on" dentistry with conditions. I was under immense pressure not to do or say anything wrong. It really reduced my confidence and my own abilities, but over time I've grown back into a confident dentist again. I felt like a convict during the GDC hearing, everyone staring over their glasses at me. I felt out of control and nobody believed my explanations, background, or my mitigating circumstances.

My words and testimony weren't respected or accepted as credible. I felt helpless and I had to put my trust and faith in my legal team, who didn't accept my arguments and defence, but preferred to follow the case how they wanted to, from their experience. Ironic how we as clinicians are taught to listen to and respect our patients, whereas my legal team had the mindset of "we know best". Ironically, they were right and I owe them my gratitude and thanks!'

The descriptions XX shares of feelings experienced during the GDC process and in particular at the hearings show what a difficult time this is for a registrant. It is a situation that is completely alien, intimidating and threatening, not to say frightening. It also demonstrates how confused an individual can get under the pressure of a referral and a hearing. These emotions and conditions are not helpful when the person is trying to respond to the issues that have been raised. In addition, the pressure can lead to reduced mental health in even the most robust registrant. The last comment, with regard to legal teams, demonstrates that the fitness to practise process is largely unknown territory for practitioners and they need to place their faith and trust in others for whom it is more familiar, that is, their legal team. For an independent practitioner, this must be uncomfortable and hard to do.

The feelings expressed above are commonly described by those who have experienced a fitness to practise referral, particularly those who have developed insight into their case. They demonstrate the model developed by Elisabeth Kübler-Ross (1969) that I have included at the end of this chapter.

The feelings that are experienced are particularly difficult for a professional person, one who is used to being respected for their experience, skills and knowledge. It cannot be overestimated how intrinsic our profession and professionalism are to our self-image. If one is under scrutiny, our own whole being is under scrutiny. The registrant is in a position they have rarely been in, with feelings of being 'out of control' and feeling guilty and having to prove innocence.

I asked XX how they felt now, some time after their case concluded and they are back working without conditions.

'I'm a lot more observant and respectful of all professional standards. I feel the GDC is too quick to progress complaints and issues, rather than re-refer for in-house management instead.

I feel I may end up again at the GDC FTP, even for minor omissions.

I carry out defensive dentistry, meaning I don't "bend over backwards" for patients any longer, and offer additional and/or extra value and service. I don't and won't risk my registration any more, even for nice patients.

I feel ashamed and embarrassed discussing my GDC history with fellow dentists. I feel scared and under pressure whenever I write up my dental notes for patients. Always double checking, even for innocent/ unintentional mistakes in grammar, as a GDC barrister could misconstrue them. I spend more time writing up thorough dental records, as it's my only defence. I've learnt it's irrelevant if the patient is happy or content with the level of service and care I offer, as it's ignored at the GDC, and they only focus on underperformance according to your record cards. I'm concerned it's so easy to make an issue over any dental records and re-refer me/anyone to the GDC – it's subjective and as we're human we're going to underperform slightly every day.'

There are many useful lessons to be learnt here and perhaps ones that the profession is being denied. I am not aware of feedback that is gathered from registrants who have concluded the fitness to practise process. This case study demonstrates positive aspects, for example a greater respect and observance of professional standards; greater regard for completion of patient records. However, there are also negative aspects: the balance of a registrant's care for their patients is ignored, the focus is on index cases, the feelings of shame and embarrassment a referred registrant feels which can prevent open discussion with colleagues. This prevents others in the profession from learning. Finally, and perhaps the saddest comment, is the practice of defensive dentistry, interpreted as a reduced willingness to 'go the extra mile'. For me, that demonstrates an erosion of the professional's core, the lasting damage, an unintended consequence that impacts on the individual, their patients, their colleagues and the wider profession.

I asked what advice XX would give to someone else going through the GDC process.

- 'Instruct an experienced legal team and expert witness who respects your strategy and follows your instructions, rather than one that think they know it all.

- Get a mentor, workplace supervisor, you trust and get on with, who can vouch/testify your professional improvements, through appraisals, audits, observations and attitude tests.
- Get as many third parties (patients, dental team, deanery) to testify on your new level of professionalism and standard of dentistry.
- Keep your cool and don't get personal or blame others for your issues.
- Accept responsibility and try to show a demarcation – that was then and this is now. You're a different dentist now, in mind, body and soul.
- Practise your answers to difficult questions and be conscious of your body language and how you come across to others.
- It's amazing coming out of the other end in June 2014; you're a new, improved and more cautious dentist. Not necessarily better, but it does focus your mind on the importance of understanding professional standards and regulatory law.
- All dentists should prepare for a GDC hearing, as statistically, unfortunately your time will come!'

These are the words of a registrant who has undergone a referral to the GDC and experienced more than one fitness to practise hearing over time as their case progressed. They worked through the conditions imposed on their practice of dentistry. They improved their working practices and worked hard to embed the changes required and provide the evidence needed by the GDC to reassure the regulator that the issues that had led to their referral would not be repeated. Only someone who has experienced this first hand can really know what it is like both professionally and personally.

For those who are referred to the GDC, the support they receive from colleagues, friends, family and professional groups can be invaluable and sometimes makes the difference between coping and not coping. These are the people and groups that XX found support from (the list is not in a particular order).

- Postgraduate dental deanery
- Indemnity organisation
- Independent paid mentors who support dentists in difficulty
- Friends and family
- Music and my faith helped me take my mind off the continual stress

A referral to the GDC is almost always a stressful experience and one that can affect the health of even the most resilient, robust individual. When I asked XX if they felt their health had suffered, this is how they responded.

'Yes definitely. I was stressed all the time, under the spotlight, working under professional GDC conditions is horrible as if "walking on egg shells", and you can't speak your mind even if you see worse dentistry and professionalism carried out around you, as I'm the one with conditions, not them!

I lost weight. I was irritable, snappy, would lose my temper quickly with my family over silly/stupid things. Other days I was introverted, didn't want to talk to anybody, just focusing on my CPD.

I felt mentally tired and exhausted, couldn't sleep, couldn't breathe calmly, I was irritable, snappy, paranoid, overthinking/analysing, I turned pessimistic rather than optimistic.

I was offered antidepressants and counselling from my GMP, but I declined.'

The health of those registrants who are referred to the GDC is not generally commented upon and yet it can have a huge impact on the ability of the person to actively respond to the referral, prepare the documents required, engage with their indemnity organisation and legal team. The personal impact on the family of those referred can be considerable. Breakdown of personal relationships is not uncommon and this at a time when the registrant is at their lowest ebb. XX noted that their mental health suffered although they soldiered on. The Dentists' Health Support Trust offers help to dental professionals who are suffering with mental health issues, substance or alcohol abuse. See Chapter 5 for more information.

Sometimes colleagues are unaware that someone in the practice has been referred to the GDC. As XX noted, there can be professional shame in being referred and an unwillingness to talk to colleagues about the referral. Most colleagues are supportive of those who are referred, although not all. This can be dependent on the case, the reasons for the referral and any part played by the practice or employing organisation.

I am indebted to XX for generously and authentically sharing their experience with the intention of helping others who might become the subject of a fitness to practise hearing. It cannot have been a comfortable thing to do and what is evident to me is how fresh the experience remains some years after the process was completed.

Case study 2: general dental practitioner (known as YY)

YY received notification from the GDC about a complaint against them in May 2009; the case was formally concluded in April 2012, just under 3 years later. Following the conclusion, YY had a published warning on their record for another 18 months. As previously, the words are those of YY and I have added my personal comments in italics.

The allegations made against YY were:
- failure to adhere to cross-infection control procedures
- failure to have indemnity cover from September 2009 until January 2011
- failure to ensure that they were vaccinated against hepatitis B whilst carrying out exposure-prone procedures
- failure to ensure good standards of clinical care as outlined in an NCAS report.

What was the GDC panel determination?

YY's case was referred to the Interim Orders Committee in February 2011 where their registration was suspended for 18 months and a referral made to the Investigating Committee, which heard the case in May 2011. At this hearing, the suspension was revoked and replaced with the following conditions.

1. Inform the GDC of any post I accept and the PCT on any performers list that I may be included on.
2. Give the GDC contact details of any employer.
3. Inform the GDC of any formal disciplinary proceedings that may be taken against me.
4. Inform the GDC if I seek employment outside the UK.
5. I must confine my practice to NHS posts under the supervision of a named dentist nominated by the local deanery.
6. I must work at the same practice as my supervisor.
7. I must have a report from my supervisor to present to the review committee.
8. I must inform within 1 week any prospective employer, locum agency or PCT on whose performers list I am seeking inclusion.
9. I must permit the GDC to disclose the above conditions to any person requesting information about my registration status.

At an Investigating Committee hearing in April 2012, the conditions were revoked and replaced by a published warning until October 2013. These were the recommendations.

1. To ensure that my PDP is up to date and reflects all learning and development needs.
2. To ensure that I work within all current and relevant guidance and professional standards.
3. To ensure that I work within all relevant guidance with regard to team working and maintain professional skills.
4. To continue for as long as necessary ongoing mentoring and coaching.

YY said that they felt 'extremely anxious and stressed' during the GDC process. At the time when I was collecting data, YY said they were feeling 'fine now'.

YY's advice to someone else going through the GDC process is:
- get as much help as possible
- recognise the mistakes that have led to the GDC referral
- be determined to correct the omissions and criticisms about your practice.

Where/who did you get support from?
Firstly, friends and family (I was supported at GDC hearings by my wife and a friend). Work colleagues, the deanery (Mersey, Manchester and Yorkshire Deanery) the BDA and DPA. My dental coach and dental mentor.

Do you feel your health suffered?
No.

Case study 3: general dental practitioner (known as ZZ)

I knew that I had developed a serious problem with dependence on alcohol. Although I never drank at work, the effects of frequent hangovers and absences from the practice were beginning to have adverse effects. I had a practice to run, wages to pay, and trying to do enough clinical dentistry during the times I was fit to work, debts were piling up, adding to the temptation to drink more to blot it all out. I couldn't see how I could take the time off to do what I knew that I should do, which was to go into rehab to help me stop drinking and deal with my problems constructively.

Things came to a head when I got a conviction for drink-driving. Fortunately, I had only got just round the corner from home, and neither I or anyone else was damaged, but a fine and a driving ban was the uncomfortable outcome. I was aware that this would probably be reported to the GDC.

I had tried to get help prior to this, but could not stop drinking for more than a few days. I finally went into rehab, a small facility for doctors and dentists in Maidenhead, where I spent Christmas and New Year. I was advised that the conviction had been picked up by the GDC, and that it would be decided the following March whether I would be referred to the Health Committee.

I spent 6 weeks in rehab, and because of my obvious efforts to get better, I had a great deal of support. My staff stayed with me, the bank manager gave me a second chance, and I was able to admit that I had been struggling, but keeping it a secret. I had entered into an Individual Voluntary Agreement (IVA) to help me to recover financially as otherwise bankruptcy would have been the only way out. losing the practice and my house very publicly.

I approached the Benevolent Fund to see if they could assist. I was, at the time, a dentist with a high profile within the profession, being a long-standing member of the GDC myself, and the Fund helped out with my rehab costs and 2 months' wages for my staff.

When I reached the Health Committee hearing, I had been clean and sober for 3 months, but I knew in my heart that I was still vulnerable. Recovery from alcohol dependence is not just about stopping drinking. The issues which started the problem in the first place have to be dealt with, new ways of dealing with anxiety and depression have to be found, life changes made.

I was given conditions which were tailored to help me to continue with recovery, but with stringent supervision. If I broke any of those conditions, then I could have been suspended from the register.

Although the quasi-judicial process was not pleasant, I viewed this as a chance to get my life back. If I wanted to keep my family, friends, staff, home and business then I had to comply with abstaining from alcohol for 3 years under the supervision of a consultant addiction specialist.

Thoughts on the GDC process
The GMC does things differently; it has a preliminary screening process where there is an option to have conditions imposed prior to a Health Committee referral. This is carried out by medically qualified personnel.

This leads to fewer Health Committee hearings but gives a doctor the opportunity to show that they are taking steps to recover (such as going into rehab) and don't pose a danger to the public.

I believe that this step is missing for dentists and there are people who are not being helped who would benefit from this approach, rather than going directly to a process that risks their registration.

The conditions given in my time were taken from a menu, and left little room for flexibility.

All were given the condition to go to a Doctors and Dentists Group, which are heavily biased towards doctors, follow the 12-Step model and have not changed in many years.

All were mandated to attend Alcoholics Anonymous (AA) meetings for 3 years. There is no requirement at such meetings for anyone to record attendance. There is a body of evidence to suggest that the success rate of this approach is low. It does not suit some people and there are now alternatives.

Do you think that your patients were at risk?
The answer to that must be yes. I would cancel appointments frequently which inconvenienced them, that of course affected the practice's financial viability. My work standards undoubtedly took a drop although there was no physical damage to anyone, and although not taking alcohol at work, I was often not really fit enough to be working and avoided doing anything but simple procedures. My staff stayed, I think, because I was a good and gener-ous employer. I wanted to do things well and I valued them as essential to the success of the business. They knew what was wrong and must have been affected by the uncertainty.

What lessons can you pass on to others?
Dental practice can be very isolating even when working in a group. We have high expectations of ourselves and so do our patients. It is very easy to imagine

that no one else experiences the same sort of problems and that everyone else is perfect. One of these expectations is that we must soldier on come what may, and admitting to a need for help is a weakness. It helps to find sources of support as soon as you admit to yourself that using alcohol or drugs is becoming problematic. This could be a supportive friend, relative or someone in your dental professional network who you trust; going to your GP should also be considered.

There is help available through the Dentists' Health Support Trust, the Practitioner's Health programme (if you live and/or work in London), and also through easily available peer support from online communities. Despite its shortcomings, there are many Alcoholics Anonymous meetings available for support in the early days. For me, it was an enormous relief not to have to hide things any more. Once people around me saw that I was serious about recovery, I was helped through the difficult early days of getting sober.

A number of years on from these events, my sobriety has been maintained and I got my life back.

Case study 4: general dental practitioner

This case study highlights the part played by the emotional state of the individual and how that can sap the ability to perform to an acceptable standard.

This was brought home to me when I worked with a registrar who was investigated by the GDC. The patient who made the complaint required an intervention needing a number of visits to be satisfactorily completed. The patient insisted that the treatment be completed more quickly. They stated they could not take off more time to complete the required number of visits the dentist said were needed. The patient pushed and pushed until the dentist complied with the pressure. The treatment did not go well and the patient complained to the GDC. As I coached the registrar, it became clear that their domestic life was by no means stable. An adult child living in another country was ill and the dentist needed to attend court hearings outside the UK to take custody of the grandchildren. She was worried sick about her daughter and grandchildren. She was in a fragile emotional state and her resilience was low. She knew she should not have agreed to undertake the treatment but her ability to resist the patient was reduced.

The case illustrates how emotional stress and anxiety can adversely affect a dental professional's ability to cope with the day-to-day pressures of practice. It also illustrates the dangers of capitulating to demands from patients that can compromise care.

Stages of change or grief

'Any natural, normal human being, when faced with any kind of loss, will go from shock all the way through acceptance.' (Kübler-Ross and Kessler, 1969)

Elisabeth Kübler-Ross was a doctor who was born in Zurich in 1926. She worked in the support and counselling of patients with personal trauma, grief and grieving associated with death and dying. She devised a model originally related to grief, but which can be used for change and emotional upset (Figure 7.3). For me, the model chimes with the upset and change that a dental professional feels during a referral to the GDC.

1. *Denial*: the change begins and the person refuses to accept the facts as presented to them. Kübler-Ross described this as a defence mechanism and a natural reaction. This is the point when a dental professional receives the initial letter from the GDC indicating that a complaint has been placed and it will be investigated. Information is requested.
2. *Anger*: the feelings of anger can be directed in a number of ways. This may be towards the person who made the complaint, towards the GDC, towards colleagues, or those closest or indeed internally towards oneself. These feelings can remain for some time and block moving on. They may also resurface at a later stage in the cycle.
3. *Bargaining*: at this stage the individual tries to seek a compromise. The bargaining can either be with another person or organisation or with themselves – 'if I do this then that will happen'.
4. *Depression*: this is where reality sinks in and often the individual can feel helpless in their ability to cope with the change, particularly as it may seem to be not of their making.
5. *Acceptance*: finally, at this stage, the person is able to accept the change.

Now that I have described the original model, I'm going to relate the five stages to the fitness to practise process. I have extended the model and added determination as a sixth stage. Over the years as I have worked with colleagues who have experienced performance difficulties, I have noticed that those who demonstrate a real and sincere determination to use the referral as a wake-up call to improve their practice are more likely not only to survive, but thrive. That is not to deny that they found the process very challenging and difficult and at times they have despaired, but their determination to learn, improve and be a better practitioner shone through.

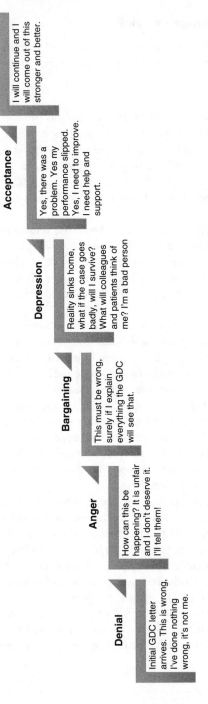

Figure 7.3 The steps of change. Applying the Kübler-Ross model to the GDC fitness to practise process (determination step added by J. A. Brooks).

Taking a preventive approach

I wrote in Chapter 1 that most dental professionals will experience a dip in their performance at some stage during their working career. I believe it is inevitable given the number of patients seen and the number of interventions dental professionals undertake. Dental professionals are human beings who suffer the same trials and tribulations as everyone else in society, with the additional stress of dentistry practice. However, measures can be taken to minimise the likelihood and severity of dips in performance whilst maximising recovery and the ability to get back to the right track.

Below is a short list of preventive actions that can reduce the risk of entering the poor performance or fitness to practise arena.

- Be aware that dips can happen.
- Take steps to not be professionally isolated – develop your network (face to face as often as possible). Take part in dentistry, in your surgery, clinic, organisation, profession.
- Keep up to date with basic aspects of dentistry as well as the more enticing, exciting aspects.
- Keep an up-to-date, dynamic PDP that you review regularly and refresh annually.
- Work with a mentor or coach or both.
- Reflect regularly on what you do, preferably with your mentor or a trusted colleague.
- Work on your communication skills as well as your clinical skills. A patient is more likely to complain if your communication is poor.
- Get to know yourself really well. Develop your self-awareness and insight and keep working on it.
- Keep healthy.
- Only undertake interventions within your scope of practice.
- Only undertake new interventions once training has been acquired.
- Keep up to date with new standards and guidance produced by the GDC, Royal Colleges, NICE and CQC.
- Undertake regular audit.
- Take part in appraisal.

There is no absolute guarantee that these actions will ensure that a dental professional will always perform well; errors and mistakes are inherent in human interactions. However, the likelihood of serious errors resulting in a complaint escalating outside the practice is reduced. In addition, when errors or mistakes do occur, they can be dealt with positively and as a means of improving future performance.

References

Campbell, J. (2014) *The Hero's Journey. Joseph Campbell on His Life and Work.* New World Library, Novato.

Cather, W. (1913) *O Pioneers.* Boston, New York

General Dental Council (GDC) (2016) *Guidelines for Whistleblowers.* General Dental Council, London.

Kübler-Ross, E. and Kessler, D. (1969) *On Grief and Grieving. Finding the Meaning of Grief Through the Five Stages of Loss.* Scribner, New York.

Vogler, C. (1992) *The Writer's Journey. Mythic Structures for Writers.* Michael Wiese Productions, Studio City, CA.

Resources

Alcoholics Anonymous www.alcoholics-anonymous.org.uk

Dentists' Health Support Trust www.dentistshealthsupporttrust.org

Life Ring Secular Recovery is an abstinence-based worldwide network. It offers peer-to-peer support to encourage personal growth and development in recovery by empowering one's 'sober self' www.LifeRing.org

Soberistas, an online community for women who are trying to get and stay sober www.Soberistas.com

Smart Recovery: learning to live life sober without reliance on 'higher powers' based on the principles of CBT. Many useful resources and online communities www.smartrecovery.org

Chapter 8 **Building self-awareness and insight**

In this chapter, I'm going to explore insight and self-awareness and the role they play in the context of performance. In addition, I will include commonly used techniques that help with deepening self-awareness and insight. Finally, I will include some tools and techniques that may be less well known that can help to deepen self-awareness and insight.

Self-awareness and insight are crucial to how dental professionals perform and behave. Those with high self-awareness and insight are less likely to sink into the mire of seriously poor performance because they can recognise the signs early and put in place ways to get back onto the right road. Those whose self-awareness and insight are not well developed can more easily get into difficulties almost without realising it until they are stuck fast.

Self-awareness and insight are powerful advantages when making change. If there is one thing that is crucial to performance, it is the ability to know when change is needed, to actually make change and to sustain change. I will add a note of caution here – that ill health can upset an individual's ability to be self-aware and insightful. If a dental professional is unwell, whether that be triggered by a physical, mental or substance cause, they are less likely to be able to recognise when performance is slipping and less able to put into place methods to get back on track. Restoring health is the priority before self-awareness and insight can be accurately assessed.

The instruments, methods and tools in this chapter are useful to all dental professionals, whether they are struggling or not. Using them can help to move good performance to great performance and help those who struggle to develop the strategies they need to turn their performance around. Finally, those who support other dental professionals can learn more about ways to support colleagues even better.

I will begin with dictionary definitions (*Oxford English Reference Dictionary*, 2nd edn, 1996).

- **Insight**: The capacity of understanding hidden truths, especially of character or situations.
- **Self-awareness**: Conscious of one's character, feelings and motives.

How to Survive Dental Performance Difficulties, First Edition. Janine Brooks.
© 2018 John Wiley & Sons Ltd. Published 2018 by John Wiley & Sons Ltd.

These two definitions are useful, but further interpretation is required within the context of performance. In addition, I will briefly consider how related the concepts are as they are often used interchangeably and rather loosely, which is not helpful.

Self-awareness and insight are complex and complicated concepts that are neither easy to define nor demonstrate. Whilst insight and self-awareness are often related and sometimes used inaccurately, they are not the same. They can be related and affect each other but it is possible to have a considerable degree of one without the other. Taken separately, they are also layered concepts; for example, a person can have insight into events and situations but have little insight into other people. In addition, self-awareness can be highly developed but faulty. For example, an individual may consider they know themselves really well and believe themselves to possess worthy qualities, but others perceive them in a different light.

Self-awareness

To possess self-awareness is to have the ability to know yourself honestly and without self-delusion. Those with good self-awareness have a clear under-standing of their own character, their strengths, weaknesses, beliefs, motivations and emotions. It is not always a comfortable talent to possess, because to be insightful means being honest with yourself. No one likes to feel they are not doing well at something. It is often easier to ignore our failings. There are also those who actually believe they are excellent at what they do, all the time. They wilfully ignore their failures, sometimes even blaming others. These are the individuals with faulty self-awareness. Healthy self-awareness is knowing yourself well, knowing your strengths, weaknesses and challenges. Appreciating that there will be times when you miss the target and being honest with yourself that you need to try harder. Self-awareness may be different to how others perceive an individual. Certain character traits, for example arrogance, can distort the lens of self-awareness.

Self-awareness is a key component of emotional intelligence. Daniel Goleman (1996) notes that self-awareness is composed of three aspects.

- Emotional awareness
- Accurate self-assessment
- Self-confidence

Being self-aware does not automatically mean you have insight. However, good self-awareness helps in understanding others and how they perceive you.

Insight

To have insight means to know where you fit with the rest of the world, how you affect those people and situations around you. To possess insight is to be able to look behind or underneath what is in front of you. An insightful

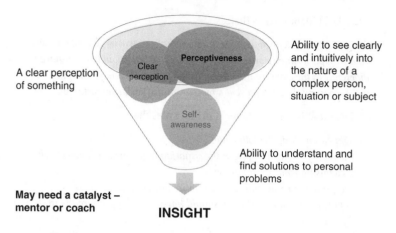

Figure 8.1 Ingredients for insight.

person will probe to find out more about a situation to more fully understand what led up to it. They will wish to understand the impact of what they do or say on others around them. In Figure 8.1, I have brought together three ingredients that I feel are important factors to develop insight. They are the ability to be perceptive; having a clear perception of a particular situation and then personal self-awareness. Together they underpin actions and the behaviours a person demonstrates to a given set of circumstances.

I believe that insight has a number of layers which include self, people, situations and events. I also believe that an individual can display good insight into one of those layers whilst having little or no insight into others. In addition, insight into impact on self and other people requires emotional intelligence that may not need to be present when being insightful about situations or events. A dental professional lacking insight would rarely question events; they would take them at face value. They would be unable to anlayse information from interactions and draw conclusions. Insight is an understanding of the impact of what you do and how that affects those around you. However, identifying, understanding and accepting that there are problems is only the first stage; an individual with well-developed insight also shows a willingness to do something about it, to improve whatever has been identified as not good enough.

> 'A readiness to explore intellectually and emotionally how and why
> I and those I interact with behave, think and feel as we do and for me to
> adapt my behaviour accordingly (insight).'
>
> *(NCAS, 2013)*

I like this definition as it draws out the dimensions of insight that go beyond self to the impact we have on others, understanding that impact, then being able to change. Our ability to be truly insightful can falter at any one of those stages.

The GDC (2016a) writes that:

'Insight might be defined as an expectation that you will be able to: review your own performance or conduct; recognise that you should have behaved differently in the circumstances being considered; and identify and put in place measures that will prevent a reoccurrence of such circumstances.'

The GDC *Case Examiner Manual* (2016a) notes that:

'Insight can include the following:
- *The ability to step back from the situation and consider it objectively;*
- *Recognising what went wrong;*
- *Accepting your role and responsibilities at the material time;*
- *Appreciating what could and should have been done differently in the circumstances;*
- *Evidencing what measures you have put into place since the allegations to avoid risk or reoccurrence; and*
- *Demonstrating how you would act differently in the future to avoid reoccurrence of a similar situation.'*

For me, the GDC definition and the *Case Examiner Manual* are more closely related to self-awareness than insight.

Kruger and Dunning (1999) highlighted that there were problems with expecting individuals to have self-insight. They noted that:'Poorly performing people (whether their performance is in the social or intellectual domain) cannot be expected to recognise their ineptitude'.

Why are poorly performing people unable to demonstrate self-insight? Because they don't know what they don't know! Expecting anyone (competent or incompetent) to assess their own performance with any degree of accuracy is very difficult. One solution would be to work with a mentor or coach who can help you test and develop your knowledge of yourself.

Holden *et al.* (2012) report that isolation and lack of insight are key features of doctors whose performance may be seriously deficient.

When assessing the degree of insight that an individual has, the following aspects of their behaviour may give clues.
- 'It's not me, it's them.'
- 'Let's get this over – how hard can it be?'
- 'I'm a good clinician – I don't see the need for all this paperwork.'
- 'I'll tell 'em.'
- Could be resistant to engage.
- Agree to everything – and do nothing.

Insight is not usually an all-or-nothing concept; dental professionals can have partial insight. The good news is that individuals can work to improve their insight.

One way to think about both self-awareness and insight is that each is composed of a number of building blocks, which are constructed of many aspects of character and are not single traits. An example of a building block would be interpersonal skills. A dental professional may be insightful about the impact they have on patients, and realise that this impact is not the one they would wish to have, but they lack or have poorly developed interpersonal skills to enable them to correct the issue. Of course, having self-awareness or insight or both does not mean that you will always act in a good way, or be ethical in your dealings with people and the world in general.

Having considered the concepts of self-awareness and insight, I now want to look at some tools that can help to increase both self-awareness and insight. However, before that and to help you consider the best tools and techniques for you, I have given an outline of different learning styles.

Learning styles

If you finished your primary dental training a few years ago, you may not have been introduced to learning styles, I know I wasn't. Back then (in the early 1980s) little thought was given to the ways individuals like to learn and what methods might work better for some people and not others. These days, there is much greater awareness of learning styles. Even so, you may not have heard of some of the work out there. Probably one of the most well-known models for learning styles is that developed by Honey and Mumford (1982).

Peter Honey and Alan Mumford developed their model using four different learning styles or ways of learning: Activist, Reflector, Theorist and Pragmatist. Their work builds on that of Kolb (1984). David Kolb, an American educational theorist, developed work on experiential learning and the idea that people learn through discovery and experience. Most people have a preference for a particular style, but are comfortable using others. Really effective learners are able to learn in all four styles. Once a person understands what their preferences are and how the other styles work, they can begin to strengthen the styles they are less comfortable with. In broad terms, Activists and Pragmatists tend to be 'doers' whilst Theorists and Reflectors tend to be 'thinkers'. It would be most unusual to find a person who demonstrated a 100% preference for only one style; most people show a preference for at least two styles. With knowledge and practice we can all improve our least favoured styles.

The styles are guides to the ways in which people like to learn. Preferences will be strengths, whereas the other styles will need more work on the part of the individual. However, a person can train themselves to develop the styles they are less strong on – the challenges. Learning preferences are not fixed in stone and everyone can work on their least well-developed preferences.

The way learning is constructed differs; there are books with text, diagrams, lectures to attend, hands-on courses, case study discussions, simulations and lots more. Some ways of learning are more strongly aligned to learning preferences than others. If the learning activity a person undertakes matches the style they prefer then their learning will be quicker. For example, if a person prefers an Activist style and attends a hands-on training course, they are more likely to learn faster. If an Activist attends a large group lecture they are likely to learn less quickly. Matching style preferences with teaching methods enhances learning. As you get to know your own learning styles and preferences, you can choose the learning format that suits you best. You are more likely to enjoy the learning and to progress much faster.

Activist (I'll try anything once)

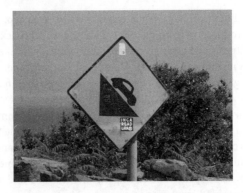

Activist learners are doers, they love new, practical experiences and like to be practical and hands on (Table 8.1). The activities they particularly like when

Table 8.1 Strengths and challenges for Activists.

Strengths	Challenges
Flexible, open-minded	Can take action without thinking
Happy to have a go	Unnecessary risks
Happy to be in new situations	Hogs the limelight
Optimistic, usually like change	Rushes into action
	Gets bored quickly

learning are group discussions and problem solving. This is the type of learner that 'has a go'; they build on what they do, improving until they get it right.

Activists are open-minded and enthusiastic about new ideas but get bored with implementation. They enjoy doing things and tend to act first and consider the implications afterwards. They like working with others but tend to hog the limelight.

Theorist (does it make sense?)

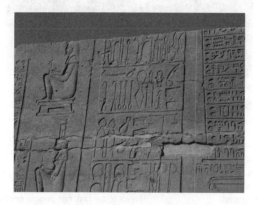

The Theorist learner likes to know what underpins the actions they take. They like to dissect and analyse. The activities that help them learn are using data and models and getting background information (Table 8.2).

Theorists adapt and integrate observations into complex and logically sound theories. They think problems through step by step. They tend to be perfectionists who like to fit things into a rational scheme. They are more likely to be detached and analytical rather than subjective or emotive in their thinking.

Table 8.2 Strengths and challenges for Theorists.

Strengths	Challenges
Logical thinker	Not a creative thinker
Rational and objective	Low tolerance for uncertainty, disorder, ambiguity
Good at asking probing questions	Intolerant of intuition and subjective
Disciplined approach	Full of oughts, musts and shoulds

Pragmatist (there's always a better way)

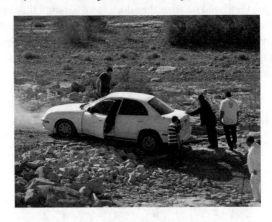

Table 8.3 Strengths and challenges for Pragmatists.

Strengths	Challenges
Keen to test out in practice	Not very interested in theory
Practical, down to earth, realistic	Tends to take first solution to a problem
Gets straight to the point	Impatient with 'waffle'
Technique orientated	Tends to be task not people orientated

Pragmatists are keen to try things out. They want concepts that can be applied to their job. They tend to be impatient with lengthy discussions and are practical and down-to-earth people (Table 8.3).

Reflector (let's not dive in, let's think about it)

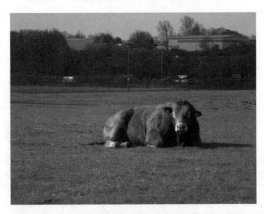

The reflective learner likes to learn by watching others and digesting what's going on. They like to look at things from a variety of angles and they like to have data. The activities that help a reflective learner learn are self-analysis and feedback from others. They also enjoy observation and shadowing others (Table 8.4).

Reflectors like to stand back and look at a situation from different perspectives. They like to collect data and think about it carefully before coming to any conclusions. They enjoy observing others and will listen to their views before offering their own.

In summary, Table 8.5 shows the activities and ways of learning that each style loves and loathes.

As you can see, one person's ideal learning situation is another's nightmare. Activists get a real buzz from lots of diverse things to get stuck into, chopping and changing, getting involved, perhaps making presentations or chairing a group. A Reflector would hate doing those things; they would tend to shut down in such situations. Reflectors prefer to think carefully about

Table 8.4 Strengths and challenges for Reflectors.

Strengths	Challenges
Careful	Tendency to hold back, not participate
Thorough and methodical	Slow to make up mind, take decisions
Thoughtful	Very cautious, risk averse
Good at listening to others	Not assertive
Rarely jumps to conclusions	

Table 8.5 Learning styles – loves and loathes.

Learning style	Love	Loathe
Activist	New problems	Lectures, theory
	Role-play	Reading, writing
	Doing things – hands on	Being on your own
	Simulation	
Reflector	Watch, observe	Role-play
	Pre-research	Insufficient data
	Analyse, review	Something that needs an instant response
Theorist	Systems, models	No context or purpose
	Structured situations	High uncertainty
	Clear purpose	Superficial, no depth
Pragmatist	Linking subject to job	'Ivory tower' teachers
	Models they can emulate	No obvious reward
	Good simulations, real problems	Too much 'faffing' about

what is going on, taking a back seat, watching the group and learning from a distance. In the same vein, Pragmatists need to be able to see how what they are learning relates to what they actually do, they like to work with experts and have little time for teachers who don't practise what they preach. This is in contrast with Theorists who enjoy interesting ideas even if they can't immediately apply them.

In a nutshell:

- Activists/Pragmatists – hands-on courses, small group informal seminar style learning
- Reflectors/Theorists – formal, lecture-style learning.

I've given only a brief introduction to the work of Honey and Mumford; if you would like to explore your learning styles in more depth, you can complete a questionnaire that will help you discover your preferences (www.talentlens. co.uk/assets/lsq/downloads/learning-styles-questionnaire-80-item.pdf). A skilled mentor can support you to strengthen those styles you feel less comfortable with. That will allow you to maximise the learning from the activities you undertake. There are other models for learning styles and you might be interested to have a look at the work of Kolb (1984), Barbe and Milone (1981), Butler and Gregorc (1988) and Riechmann and Grasha (1974).

Tools to deepen self-awareness

Having introduced the idea that people learn in different ways, you might want to ponder that whilst reading about the sort of tools that can help you.

In this section I'm going to give an overview of three tools.

- Myers–Briggs Type Indicator (MBTI)
- Neuro-Linguistic Programming (NLP)
- Thomas–Kilmann Conflict Mode Instrument (TKI)

All these tools and instruments should be administered and interpreted by a trained practitioner. This is because they are quite complex and if you are to get the best out of them then they need to be properly undertaken. These are not 'self-reporting' questionnaires, which give predictions; they are well-researched, well-validated techniques. This is good news for dental professionals who generally like to know that techniques have a solid basis to them and are not 'fluffy'. I will be giving references to articles and publications that you will find helpful if you would like to delve deeper.

Myers-Briggs Type Indicator (MBTI)

The Myer-Briggs Type Indicator (MBTI) was developed from the work of Carl Jung (1875–1961), a Swiss psychiatrist and psychologist, who proposed a theory of psychological types where people are innately different, both in terms of the way they see the world and take in information, and how they make decisions. Jung's work was taken up by Katharine Briggs (1875–1968) and her daughter Isobel Myers (1897–1980) who thought his ideas were so useful that they wanted to make them accessible to a wider audience. In 1943, MBTI was launched. It is comprised of a self-report questionnaire and a guide for the person to decide their best fit to the 16 types.

MBTI identifies valuable differences between normal healthy people and it highlights differences that can be the source of misunderstanding, miscommunication and strife. It helps individuals identify their unique gifts and enhances self-awareness. In addition, it highlights natural strengths, potential areas for growth and an appreciation of the differences people display.

The indicator describes personality differences positively and there are no worse or better types, each has strengths and possible blind spots. There is good quality research into the use of the indicator including in the health services. The indicator has reliability and validity.

Our preferences tell us what we find most energising and comfortable. The type cannot determine skill or ability and should not be used for recruitment purposes. We can each use all eight preferences and the person themselves is best at deciding their own type. The types are known as:

Extraversion (E) v Introversion (I)
Sensing (S) v Intuition (N)
Thinking (T) v Feeling
Judging (J) v Perceiving (P)

It is important to think about the descriptors used in the MBTI as the terminology can at times be unhelpful.

- "Extravert" does not mean "talkative" or "loud"
- "Introvert" does not mean "shy" or "inhibited"
- "Feeling" does not mean "emotional"
- "Judging" does not mean "judgmental"
- "Perceiving" does not mean "perceptive"

The table below shows how the 16 types are made up from the eight preferences.

ISTJ	ISFJ	INFJ	INTJ
ISTP	ISFP	INFP	INTP
ESTP	ESFP	ENFP	ENTP
ESTJ	ESFJ	ENFJ	ENTJ

Being forced to work outside of your preference for any length of time can be a major source of stress. It can be particularly difficult for introverts who have to interact in an extrovert world.

Preference, as described by the Myers-Briggs instrument, can help to increase self-awareness and also to appreciate the differences between the way people like to operate. This can be extremely helpful when working with individuals. Within dentistry it can help to understand interactions between colleagues, staff and patients. It can help to reduce misunderstanding and conflict. If you wish to delve deeper into the use of Myers-Briggs it is best to work with someone trained in the use and interpretation of the preferences. They can help guide you to get the most out of your personal analysis. However, there is plenty of published work using Myers-Briggs that is interesting to read and I've included some references at the end of this chapter.

As we get older and our experience and confidence grows, usually our self-awareness deepens. As this happens we become more adept at using the non-preference aspects of type. We become more rounded.

MBTI Distribution of Types

Whilst the MBTI 16 types are found distributed across the globe they are not evenly distributed. Certain groups within the population will show more or less of particular types, for example gender.

Most of the types are distributed in a similar way between males and females with the exception of thinking and feeling. Females are more likely to demonstrate a feeling preference than males. This may be significant in the dental profession as those with a feeling preference are likely to make decisions based on values where they are guided by personal values and focus on harmony. Those with a feeling preference look for common ground and treat each person as a unique individual.

Barran (2005) looked at 202 dentists practicing in Illinois, North America using the MBTI preferences. The study, suggested that some MBTI personality types tend to be at greater risk of burnout and the negative effects of stress. The specific type of ISTJ stands out as one that responds negatively to the stressors of dental practice. Other types at risk are ISFJ and INFP.

Al-Dlaigan et al (2017) reviewed the MBTI types of 243 dental specialists working in Saudia Arabia and found that "more than 50 per cent of all specialists shared one common type of personality (ISTJ)".

As mentioned above, I recommend that you work with a trained Myers Briggs practitioner who will be able to administer the questionnaire, but more importantly work with you on the feedback and support you to discover your best-fit preferences.

Neuro-Linguistic Programming (NLP)

The beginnings of NLP can be found in the 1950s–1960s with the Human Potential movement which looked at modelling happy people (Maslow, 1962; Rogers, 1965). This work continued through the 1960s and 1970s with 'maverick thinkers' Milton Erikson (1974) and Fritz Perls (1969) and finally to the 1970s and 1980s when early NLP began to emerge. Bandler and Grinder (1979) and Dilts (1990) modelled and codified successful people and the things they did. That work was extended into the field of sport (Gallwey, 1974) and emotional intelligence (Goleman, 1996). Finally, in the 1990s NLP began to be used and known more widely.

What do the NLP words mean?

- *Neuro*: how we process the information we receive from our senses.
- *Linguistic*: the words, language and non-verbal communication we use to make sense of the information we receive.
- *Programming*: patterns of thoughts or behaviours that can help us or get in the way of what we want to achieve.

Neuro-Linguistic Programming is a process we can use to make change, a way to move from where we are now to where we want to be; you could think of it as a mode of transport to help us move from A to B.

The use of 'trans language' to change another person's state, by guidance or persuasion, is important in NLP. The use of words and language is crucial in dentistry. Using the wrong words or the right words inappropriately can make the difference between a patient complaint or compliance. Within dentistry, the impact of the language we use is not well understood. Words are the way we influence what we want others to do. If we choose the right words used in the right context and our expectation is for the other person to succeed, then they are more likely to do so. When talking to patients, if we expect the patient to succeed, perhaps by improving their tooth brushing, and we use the right words to enhance motivation then the patient is much more likely to engage and succeed. Conversely, and with particular relevance to performance, the reverse is also true. If we use the wrong words and our expectation is that the patient will fail, then that is more likely to be the result.

A model used in NLP is neurological levels; you can find more about that in Chapter 10.

Common limiting beliefs

These are beliefs that individuals may hold about themselves and life in general. Because individuals feel the belief to be true, they act in a way that can make it true. This is why these beliefs are limiting – they limit what people think is possible. The belief is often very strongly held and it may have its roots in childhood. Individuals may have learnt these beliefs because they were told them by their parents. Beliefs may have developed from an experience that was traumatic or had a long-lasting impression. Wherever and whenever they began, common limiting beliefs can wield great power and influence.

Field and Field (2014) suggest some common limiting beliefs.

- I must be loved or accepted by everyone
- I must be perfect in all I do
- All the people with whom I work or live have to be perfect
- I'm a bad person if I make a mistake
- Somewhere there is the perfect job, the perfect solution, the perfect partner, and all I need to do is search for them
- People, including me, do not change
- I should not have problems. If I do, it means I'm incompetent
- Change is always difficult and takes time

I'm sure you could add to this list, probably 10 times over. I'm also sure you recognise some of these limiting beliefs. You might want to take time to think about what the opposite belief is to any of those above. I think of those as liberating beliefs.

- People, including me, do change
- I'm not a bad person if I make a mistake
- I may have problems, but it doesn't mean I am incompetent

I've picked out three that have particular resonance for those who are struggling with their performance. Limiting beliefs can keep us in a spiral and make it very difficult to break out; they sap our ability to take control. Liberating beliefs can help us see we are in control; one mistake doesn't make us a bad person, it makes us human. Thinking about limiting beliefs with a coach can be very helpful as a coach can support their coachee to challenge the limiting belief, turn it into a liberating belief, take control and move forward positively.

Representational systems
Neuro-Linguistic Programming refers to the way we interact with the world using our senses as representational systems.

You may have come across VAK (visual, auditory, kinaesthetic). Representational systems are those that use our five senses – visual, auditory, touch, taste and olfactory. We use our senses all the time, it's the way we collect data from the world around us and our senses underpin the way we code the world and the language we use to describe it. For example, when learning something new, some of us may prefer to see it or imagine it performed, others need to hear how to do it, others need to get a feeling for it, and yet others have to make sense of it. In general, one system is not better than another and sometimes it depends on the situation or task that we are learning or doing as to which representational system might be more effective. For example, if you're painting a portrait then the visual system will be more engaged; if you're listening to an audiobook then you would be using more of your auditory system. Most of us have a preferred representational system that we use most often when we speak, communicate and learn. People at the top of their profession typically have the ability to use all the representational systems and to choose the one most appropriate for the situation.

We have five senses and they link to the representational system, as illustrated in Figure 8.2.

The VAK concept was first developed by psychologists and teaching specialists such as Keller (2014), Orton (2014), Gillingham and Stillman

Sense	Representational system	Image
Sight	Visual	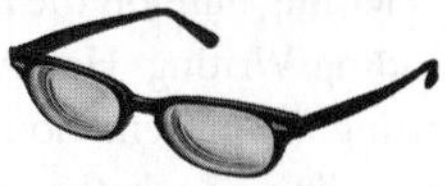
Hearing	Auditory	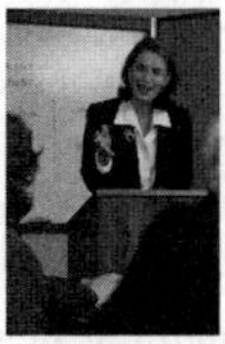
Feeling	Kinaesthetic	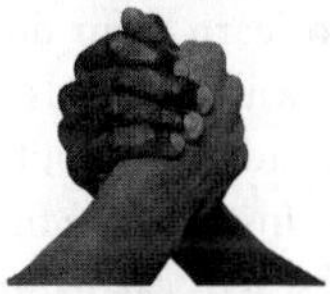
Smell	Olfactory	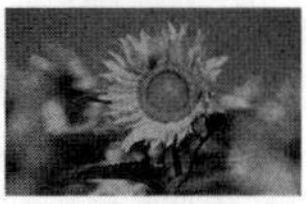
Taste	Gustatory	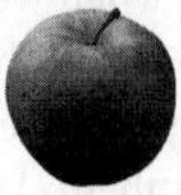

Figure 8.2 Representational systems.

Table 8.6 VAK – language mapped to the representational styles.

Visual	Auditory	Kinaesthetic
It looks like	It sounds like	It feels like
Show me what you mean	We're on the same wavelength	Solid as a rock
This is clear cut	Important to ask me	Get to grips with
Sight for sore eyes	Word for word	Pain in the neck
My perspective is	My question is	My emotional reaction is

(1997), Stillman (1928) and Montessori (1912). The VAK/VARK model was developed by Neil Fleming in 1987 (Fleming and Mills, 1992). It's an example of a representational system and expands on earlier work used in NLP (Table 8.6).

Fleming built on the model of Visual/Auditory and Kinaesthetic to add in Reading/Writing. He divided the Visual aspect, separating out reading and writing. Representational systems use the premise that we learn better depending on whether we use visual methods, for example pictures or diagrams, auditory cues or through touch or feel. Visual people will use words such as 'show me', let's have a look at that'. They like to read instructions or observe someone doing a task before they attempt it themselves. Auditory individuals like to hear information, so they enjoy learning through music, discussion or lecture presentations. They will use words such as 'tell me' or 'let's talk it over'. They like to listen to instructions from an expert before they try something new. They are also quite happy taking spoken instructions over the telephone. Then, some people with a kinaesthetic learning style prefer to learn from doing things. They like practical hands-on experiences. They will use words such as 'let me try' or 'how do you feel?'. They prefer to go ahead and try out a new experience, learning as they go. They rarely look at the instructions first.

Research carried out by Grinder and Bandler in the 1970s (Grinder and Bandler, 1976) found that people communicate more easily when they are part of a group with the same representational system rather than in groups who have mixed preferences. Some of us use all five sensory representations when we learn, but most of us tend to prefer one or two.

We can improve our communication with other people and also our own learning when we know more about their preferences and how they match our own. To do that with representational systems, we need to identify other people's preferences. We do that by listening to the words people use and how they use them. When we know which system they prefer, we can connect with them more easily. As you learn more about the systems and begin to understand yourself and the language you use, you will be able to adapt your

Table 8.7 VAK – language examples.

Task	Visual	Auditory	Kinaesthetic
Operate new equipment	Read instructions	Listen to explanation	Have a go
Travel directions	Look at a map	Ask for spoken directions	Follow your nose
Teach someone something	Write instructions	Explain verbally	Demonstrate and let them have a go
They'd say	I see what you mean Show me Watch how I do it	I hear what you are saying Tell me Listen to me explain	I know how you feel Let me try You have a go

style to match the people you are communicating with. There are obvious benefits here when talking to and listening to patients. Tables 8.6 and 8.7 give some examples of the words used by the three sensory channels: visual, auditory and kinaesthetic.

The preferences are not all or nothing and some people are equally comfortable using all three styles, but most seem to be more at home with one or two. Once you are more aware of your own style, you will begin to notice the preferences of those you work with. This is particularly noticeable in the words people use. As you become more aware, you can begin to match your learning style to what works best for you and your learning is likely to improve.

Present state to desired state
This is a way to think about moving from A (present) to B (desired). For those who are within the fitness to practise process, the present state is the regulatory process and the desired state is for the regulatory process to be concluded. To make the transition, most people will need help (resources). A number of the resources could be external to the person. NLP looks at the internal resources, sometimes thought of as states of mind or attitudes.

Perceptual positions
Work on perceptual positions was undertaken by John Grinder and Judith DeLozier in 1987. They suggest that we can look at relationships from different perceptions. There are three primary positions (Figure 8.3).
- *Self*: experience perceived from the individual's point of view, looking out at the world. Those who spend most of their time in this position can become self-absorbed and lack awareness of other people.

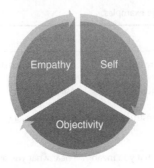

Figure 8.3 Primary perceptual positions.

- *Empathy*: looking at the world from another person's point of view. This allows information to be gained from their perspective and gives 'self' knowledge about the effect we have on the other person. Those who spend most of their time in this position can lose themselves and become disengaged from their own experiences.
- *Objectivity*: you could imagine this as a 'fly on the wall', an observer who is outside their interactions with other people. This can be a position taken when reflecting on a past interaction. Those who spend most of their time in this position can appear remote and cold to others.

Individuals who have good self-awareness and good communication skills can use all three positions rather than becoming stuck in any one. A personal development is to consider the three perceptual positions and think about whether you spend more time in one. If you do, then you have identified an area you might wish to work on and strengthen your use of the underused positions.

Thomas–Kilmann Conflict Mode Instrument (TKI)

This instrument was developed by Kenneth Thomas and Ralph Kilmann in the early 1970s. It is based on a model of managerial conflict styles introduced by Blake and Mouton (1964). Thomas and Kilmann initially developed the instrument as a research tool. I find it helpful to understand responses to stress and conflict and how those responses can enable or disable individuals to cope, learn from their experiences and work through difficult situations. For dental professionals, there are few more difficult situations than those presented by performance concerns and regulation. The stress and potential mental conflict that arise from a complaint, the investigation, referral to the commissioner or the GDC are considerable.

I'm going to use the TKI as a model to help in understanding different ways of reacting to the stress and conflict that can be part of poor performance. Knowing more about the ways that individuals prefer to react can help in learning which ways can be most successful, when each way might be best and what skills are needed to use each mode. All the modes are useful and effective, but when used in relation to performance, some are likely to be more effective than others and some can lead to an escalation of the issue, thus reducing the chance of a good outcome for the practitioner.

The TKI can be administered and interpreted by most Myers–Briggs practitioners. It is wise to work with someone skilled in its use to maximise your knowledge of how you approach conflict/stressful situations. As with the majority of tools that can help increase self-awareness, there is no right, wrong or perfect mode. All five are useful in certain situations and less useful in others. What is important is using the right mode for the right situation and how skilful you are in utilising a specific mode.

The TKI suggests there are two core ways (or dimensions) in which individuals choose to react to a conflict situation; assertiveness or co-operativeness. In the context of poor performance, the conflict can be viewed as how an individual handles the stress of a complaint or a referral to the regulator. In the TKI, the two dimensions are separate and are not considered to be opposites of each other. So a person can be both assertive and co-operative, you don't have to be either/or.

- *Assertiveness*: this illustrates how much an individual seeks to satisfy their own concerns or how much they want to get support for their ideas.
- *Co-operativeness*: this shows how much an individual seeks to satisfy other people's concerns or how receptive they are to other people's ideas.

The two dimensions can be depicted as the two axes of a graph.

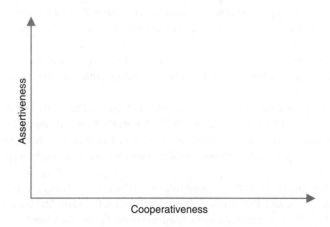

The TKI then adds five ways of handling conflict (Figure 8.4). These illustrate the behaviours that individuals demonstrate when reacting to a conflict

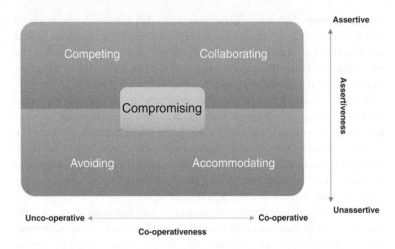

Figure 8.4 TKI modes of seeking resolution.

situation. They combine assertiveness and co-operativeness with varying emphasis on the two dimensions.

The diagram depicts the five different ways (or modes) of seeking resolution; they should not be confused with the behaviours that individuals display when using each mode. I'll briefly look at each in turn then consider how they relate to ways of handling the conflict that can arise when there is a performance concern (Table 8.8).

- *Competing*: this combines the dimensions of assertive and unco-operative. An individual who competes likes to satisfy their concerns at the expense of others.
- *Collaborating*: this combines assertion with co-operation. An individual who collaborates tries to find a solution that satisfies everyone's concerns.
- *Compromising*: this is a middle-of-the-road position between the two dimensions of assertiveness and co-operativeness. It aims to find a position acceptable to both, but only partially succeeds. Any compromise is just that – no one person feels they have achieved what they wanted.
- *Avoiding*: This is neither assertive nor co-operative. This position hopes that if the situation is ignored, it will go away. Ultimately, this tends to just delay the inevitable and can sometimes make the position worse.
- *Accommodating*: the person who tries to be accommodating is unassertive yet co-operative. They hope that by addressing the other person's issues, the problem will be solved. They do this at the expense of what they wish to achieve.

Table 8.8 TKI modes, relationship to dental performance.

Mode	Relationship to dental performance
Competing	An individual that uses this way of handling a complaint may try to impose their authority. They often believe they are right and everyone else is wrong; this includes the patient, their staff and the GDC. They may try to brow beat or demean the other party. They will try to find a resolution that fits their agenda and their way of looking at events. As a mode of operating, this rarely ends well
Collaborating	The Collaborating individual tries to combine the insights they discover into a better understanding. They will often be able to see both sides of an argument or concern and want to work to resolve the situation for everyone. In addition, they are often keen to improve the outcome. These people take the lemons that come from a complaint and turn them into lemonade. They will turn a difficult situation into a future that is better than the reality before the complaint
Compromising	A person who uses this method will try to find the middle road for everyone. Unfortunately, this can often lead to one party (or sometimes both) feeling they have given more than they have taken and dissatisfaction is the result
Avoiding	Avoiding is a common method, particularly by those who do not like conflict and confrontation. An example would be a member of staff who is frequently late. Often the person who should take action does not because they do not want an argument. they leave it, hoping the situation will resolve itself
Accommodating	The Accommodating person when faced with a member of staff who is frequently late would try to alter working practices to allow the late comer to begin their work later. This may work, but the result may be that the later comer is even later

Each mode is useful when used in the right situation with the right skills. Not all are appropriate when reacting to the stress of a performance investigation; some have more costs than benefits for that situation (Table 8.9).

You can see that each of these modes of operating when working with others could be more or less successful, depending on the situation. All can be helpful at times and unhelpful at others. As you know more about the modes, you can put them to good use in your everyday interactions with other people. Used successfully and skilfully, they can reduce the potential for misunderstandings and complaint. You can learn the skills you need to increase the benefits of each mode and reduce the costs. You can learn to avoid an issue without appearing evasive or compete without others becoming angry.

When dealing with and reacting to the stress of performance issues, some modes are more successful than others. Table 8.10 looks at which are most useful (and which to avoid). In addition, I have indicated the skills you may wish to develop or strengthen.

Table 8.9 TKI modes – benefits and costs of each mode.

Mode	Benefits	Costs	Notes
Competing	Standing up for yourself Pushing for a quick decision Protecting your interests	Other person may feel resentful, exploited Deadlock Can be viewed as provocative	
Collaborating	Working to meet your and others concerns, resolve conflict Exchange information freely Seeking solutions	Time consuming Individual could be exploited by the other parties Can make things worse	Helpful when working with those who will support you – indemnity, mentor, educational supervisor, deanery
Compromising	Getting a solution that is good enough Make a settlement Meeting halfway	Both parties frustrated Lower quality solution Superficial understanding, could escalate	Can be the way an indemnity organisation suggests to reduce possibility of complaint to GDC
Avoiding	Failure to engage Viewing issue as time wasting and low priority	Viewed as evasive and arrogant No learning Escalation, as there is no resolution	
Accommodating	Give the other person what they want Let sleeping dogs lie Cutting losses, move on	You lose yourself Respect is diminished Your interests are sacrificed	

Table 8.10 TKI modes – when to use and skills to develop.

Mode	When most useful	Skills to develop to be most successful
Competing	Use very occasionally, it can alienate others. For issues which are vital and when Collaborating is not feasible or appropriate. For example, if you have rock-solid evidence that you did or did not do something essential to the case	Being persuasive (without being threatening or arrogant) Being fair (this is not about beating the other side into submission) Using warnings not threats, being specific and credible Being respectful
Collaborating	Recognising the conditions that help collaboration Issues are important enough to collaborate	Interpersonal skills, communicate skilfully Openness to new ideas Integrating possibilities
Compromising	For significant issues where Competing and Collaboration are not appropriate	Insight to know when there are real concerns with your practice Humility Objective assessment of the facts
Avoiding	When to postpone an issue	Control anger Steer clear of being personal Refocusing complex and sensitive issues Know when evasive tendency raises its head
Accommodating	Yielding to the facts, when you are wrong	Learn to use complaints/feedback constructively Active listening Be graceful in accepting that you can improve

Conclusion

Having considered a number of tools that you can use to help with raising self-awareness and insight, the next chapter deals with tools you can use for personal development and building your PDP.

References

Al-Dlaigan, Y.H., Alahmari, A.S., Almubarak, S.H., Alateeq, S.A. and Anil, S. (2017) Study on personality types of dentists in different disciplines of dentistry. *Journal of Contemporary Dental Practice*, **18**(7), 554–558.

Bandler, R. and Grinder, J. (1979) *Frogs into Princes: Neuro Linguistic Programming*. Real People Press, Boulder, CO.

Baran, R.B. (2005) Myers–Briggs Type Indicator: burnout and satisfaction in Illinois dentists. *Practice Management*, 228–234.

Barbe, W.B. and Milone, M.N. (1981) What we know about modality strengths? Association for Supervision and Curriculum Development, Alexandria, VA, pp. 378–380.

Blake, R.R. and Mouton, J.S. (1964) *The Managerial Grid*. Gulf, Houston, TX.

Butler, K.A. and Gregorc, A.F. (1988) *It's All in Your Mind: A Student's Guide to Learning Style*. Learner's Dimension, Columbia, CT.

Dilts, R. (1990) *Changing Belief Systems with NLP*. Meta Publications, Capitola, CA.

Erikson, E.H. (1974) *Dimensions of a New Identity*. Jefferson Lectures in the Humanities. W.W. Norton, New York.

Field, J. and Field, S. (2014) NLP Practitioner, Module 1. Available at: www.field-field.com.

Fleming, N.D. and Mills, C. (1992) *Not Another Inventory, Rather a Catalyst for Reflection*. Available at: http://vark-learn.com/wp-content/uploads/2014/08/not_another_inventory.pdf (accessed 11 January 2018).

Gallwey, W.T. (1974) *The Inner Game of Tennis*. Random House, New York.

General Dental Council (GDC) (2016a) *Investigating Committee Guidance Manual*. General Dental Council, London, p. 26.

General Dental Council (GDC) (2016b) *Case Examiner Manual*. General Dental Council, London, p. 17.

Gillingham, A. and Stillman, B.W. (1997) *The Gillingham Manual: Remedial Training for Students with the Specific Disability in Reading, Spelling and Penmanship*, 8th edn. Educators Publishing Service, Cambridge, MA.

Goleman, D. (1996) *Emotional Intelligence. Why It Can Matter More than IQ*. Bantam Books, New York.

Grinder, J. and Bandler, R. (1976) *The Structure of Magic, Vol.* **II**. Science and Behavior Books, Palo Alto, CA.

Grinder, J. and DeLozier, J. (1987) *Turtles All the Way Down*. Metamorphous Press, Portland, OR

Holden, J.D., Cox, S.J. and Hargreaves, S. (2012) *Avoiding Isolation and Gaining Insight*. BMJ Careers. BMJ Publishing Group, London.

Honey, P. and Mumford, A. (1982) *Manual of Learning Styles*. Honey and Mumford, London.

Keller, J.M. (2014) *Motivational Design for Learning and Performance. The ARCS Model Approach*. Springer, New York.

Kolb, D.A. (1984) *Experiential Learning: Experience as the Source of Learning and Development*. Prentice-Hall, Englewood Cliffs, NJ.

Kruger, J. and Dunning, D. (1999) Unskilled and unaware of it: how difficulties in recognising one's own incompetence lead to inflated self-assessment. *Journal of Personality and Social Psychology*, **77**, 1121–1134.

Maslow, A.H. (1962) Notes on being-psychology. *Journal of Humanistic Psychology*, **2**(2), 47–71.

Montessori, M. (1912) *The Montessori Method*. Frederick A. Stoke, New York.

Myers, I.B., McCaulley, M.H., Quenk, N.L. and Hammer, A.L. (1998) *MBTI Manual: A Guide to the Development and Use of the Myers–Briggs Type Indicator*, 3rd edn. Consulting Psychologists Press, Palo Alto, CA.

National Clinical Assessment Service (2013) Defining insight – a challenge that matters. Poster v 1.1. National Clinical Assessment Service, London.

Orton, K. (2014) Reflective practice: what's the problem? *Education Today*, **64**(3), 25–30.

Perls, F. (1969) *Ego, Hunger, and Aggression: The Beginning of Gestalt Therapy*. Random House, New York.

Riechmann, S.W. and Grasha, A.F. (1974) A rational approach to developing and assessing the construct validity of a student learning style scales instrument. *Journal of Psychology*, **87** (2), 213–223.

Rogers, C.R. (1965) The place of the person in the new world of the behavioral sciences, in *Humanistic Viewpoints in Psychology: A Book of Readings* (ed. F.T. Severin). McGraw-Hill, New York, pp. 387–407.

Stillman, B.W. (1928) *Training Children to Study*. DC Heath, Boston, MA.

Chapter 9 **Tools that can help**

Having covered aspects of self-awareness and insight in the previous chapter, in this chapter I intend to describe a number of tools that will help with personal development.

The tools in this chapter are not just for those who may be struggling or who have an ongoing fitness to practise case. They are for all dental professionals. We all need to use these tools to ensure we are providing the best service we can to our patients. All the tools I have included can easily be used by any dental professional; there is nothing mystical about them and they need very little in the way of 'kit' to complete them. Some may be familiar to readers, others less so. Some you will find more useful than others, depending on what you are seeking and what aspect of your life and practice you want to improve or change.

- Personal development plan
- Peer review
- Professional discussion and dialogue
- Case studies/case presentation
- Clinical audit
- Staff meetings
- Patient surveys (feedback)
- 360° (multisource) feedback
- Standards, national guidelines
- Working with a mentor
- Working with a coach

You will notice that I haven't specifically included continuing professional development (CPD) as a bullet point. The reason is that all the activities above can be described as CPD, but not all could be termed verifiable. CPD is an umbrella term which, if undertaken positively, has a powerful effect on good patient care. In that sense, all the tools covered in this chapter constitute CPD. Verifiable CPD needs to meet particular criteria and these can be found on the GDC website. However, all these tools can provide valuable evidence for meeting determination requirements as part of GDC fitness to practise processes.

How to Survive Dental Performance Difficulties, First Edition. Janine Brooks.
© 2018 John Wiley & Sons Ltd. Published 2018 by John Wiley & Sons Ltd.

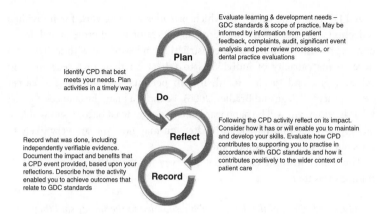

Plan

Evaluate learning & development needs – GDC standards & scope of practice. May be informed by information from patient feedback, complaints, audit, significant event analysis and peer review processes, or dental practice evaluations

Identify CPD that best meets your needs. Plan activities in a timely way

Do

Record what was done, including independently verifiable evidence. Document the impact and benefits that a CPD event provided, based upon your reflections. Describe how the activity enabled you to achieve outcomes that relate to GDC standards

Reflect

Following the CPD activity reflect on its impact. Consider how it has or will enable you to maintain and develop your skills. Evaluate how CPD contributes to supporting you to practise in accordance with GDC standards and how it contributes positively to the wider context of patient care

Record

Figure 9.1 Enhanced CPD.

Continuing professional development is an activity that all dental registrants are required to undertake to maintain their registration. The GDC prescribes how much CPD should be undertaken over a period of 5 years – the CPD cycle. There is a huge variety of CPD coupled with a wide variety of formats. As the term implies, it needs to be undertaken as a continuous part of a professional's career; there is no start or finish other than it begins when the professional qualifies and first registers with the GDC and it finishes when the professional completes their professional career and is no longer a registrant. The activity undertaken must be relevant to the registrant's professional work. Finally, the activity is concerned with development. I think of this as growth, something new or different. Of course, CPD must also include keeping up to date and maintaining knowledge and competence, so not every activity needs to be about developing new skills; revising, refreshing and renewing are important aspects of CPD. For CPD to be truly useful and effective, it should include a wide variety of activities and reflect the registrant's learning style whenever possible to maximise what is actually learned and retained.

Enhanced CPD

This was introduced on 1 January 2018 for dentists and 1 August 2018 for dental care professionals (Figure 9.1).

Personal development plan

All dental professionals must have a personal development plan (PDP). A PDP is basically a plan of how an individual will develop their skills, knowledge and outlook over a period of time. It is *not* a measure of performance and should not be used as one.

A PDP is a structured tool which provides a framework for individual reflection and action planning based on educational and professional development needs. The purpose of constructing and working with a PDP is to develop the capacity of individuals to reflect on their own learning and achievement, and to plan for their own personal educational and career development, (Clegg and Bradley, 2006). Without a plan, the chances are that your development will be haphazard and based on what becomes available at any given time. You may be fortunate, you may not. You are very likely to miss out on something important.

The Picker Institute carried out a survey for the GDC and one of their findings was that:

'Over half (55%) of the dentists who responded to the survey said they had been involved in personal development planning over the last year. Half of the respondents carried it out as part of appraisal.'

(Chisholm et al., 2012, p. 38).

The survey only included dentists and it highlighted a number of important aspects about the use of PDPs. For example, not all dental professionals in all branches of dentistry demonstrated a similar useage of PDPs. Those least likely to have a PDP are those working in:

- general dental services
- all private practice
- Scotland.

Those who are most likely to have a PDP are those working in:

- community services and hospital settings
- NHS setting
- England
- specialist practice.

A number of suggestions were given as to why these differences exist. For example, those working in community or hospital settings will generally be working in a more structured line management arrangement and performance management processes will be well established. In England, a requirement was put in place by primary care trusts (when they existed) that all principal dentists have a PDP.

So, without wishing to labour the point, a PDP is:

- *personal* – about you
- *development* – about your development
- *plan* – how you will do it (usually in the next 12–18 months).

When constructing a PDP, give thought to the following.

- Individual development needs.
- The learning activities needed to achieve the development need.

- Preferred learning styles.
- Helpers/supporters/other resources.
- Measures of achievement that can be used to evidence successful completion of the activity.
- Time limits; a PDP must always be timed, never vague as in 'the next 6 months'.
- Demonstrate how you will embed what you have learned in a way that will benefit patients.

If an activity will have no benefit to patients either directly or indirectly, then serious consideration should be given to whether it is worth undertaking. All dental professionals, no matter which aspect of dentistry they work in, are in service to patients. When I present a lecture, it is to enhance the knowledge of fellow professionals to enable them to improve the service they provide to patients. When I mentor or coach a fellow professional, it is to support them to improve how they operate within dentistry and ultimately to be better at providing a service to patients. When I work as an educational inspector for the GDC, it is to encourage the best possible educational environment for training dental professionals who will qualify to provide a service to patients.

Before writing or reviewing your PDP, it can be helpful to work through the following steps.

1. Stock-take your current skills, ability and knowledge.
2. Set objectives for what you want to achieve.
3. Identify the areas you need to develop.
4. Decide on the steps needed to close the gap (NB: remember learning style).
5. Review regularly.

When constructing a PDP, I recommend that you use the SMART format to ensure that the plan really aids your development and is not just 'window dressing'. I'm sure the format is familiar to most, but just to refresh:

S – Specific
M – Measurable
A – Achievable
R – Relevant/Realistic
T – Timely

A mentor can help to facilitate preparation and construction of a PDP. More detail about mentors and mentoring can be found later in the chapter.

The GDC requires that all registrants *must* have an active PDP. This is interesting as it takes the requirement beyond just having a PDP to having an *active* PDP. This means one that is used, is dynamic and regularly impacts on its creator.

The actual requirement is for:
- a PDP which details the CPD you plan to undertake and associated learning outcomes. This may evolve throughout your cycle
- a log of completed activity, including date, number of hours and which learning outcome it covered (GDC PC Conditions Bank, May 2014).

A final word about PDPs. If you have a portfolio career, that is, you work in more than one aspect of dentistry, you need to include development activities for each aspect. For example, if you are a training programme director, then you should include activities that will keep you up to date with educational activities.

Many of the tools included in this chapter can help in achieving aspects of your PDP and in providing evidence that you have completed an activity. There are many formats for PDPs provided by organisations within dentistry; you do not have to construct your own. An example is given at the end of this chapter in Appendix A. Please feel free to use it if it helps.

Peer review

'Peer review is the professional assessment, against standards, of the organisation of healthcare processes and quality of work, with the objective of facilitating its improvement.'

(Healthcare Foundation, 2012)

Peer review is an activity undertaken by groups of dental professionals, generally between four and eight individuals. The purpose is to review an aspect of practice, perhaps using a case or intervention, then to share the experiences of each individual within the group and finally, together to identify where change/improvement is possible. The purpose is to share in an environment of learning between colleagues – 'peers'. It is a good idea to keep notes of peer review meetings as they are formal learning activities, not just a chat with friendly colleagues. The notes should include the topic of the review, who was present, observations made and action points agreed. While a single practice can operate peer review internally, particularly a large one, it is even better to partner with another practice or practices if possible. This helps to add to the diversity of ideas and expertise within the group and makes the peer review even stronger.

Professional discussion and dialogue

Professional discussion and dialogue is a two-way planned conversation between two professionals. It can help to deepen knowledge or pass on new knowledge. The important aspects are that it is planned and two-way. It is not a chance corridor conversation or a snatched 5-minute catch-up. The two people need to find dedicated, uninterrupted time in a quiet space; 30 minutes is probably a good amount of discussion time. The topic(s) for discussion should be agreed ahead of the conversation so that the discussion is focused and does not slide into a 'happy chat'.

The activity works well with trainees and new members of the team.

Group professional discussion and dialogue is a variation. Here, a group of dental professionals agree the topic(s) they wish to discuss, for example a particular intervention or condition. One person is asked to lead or chair the discussion to keep focus and prevent side tracking. It is probably best to keep the discussion to no more than 1 hour. Whilst most people may like the discussion to be face to face, use of Skype or Facetime can also work provided everyone is comfortable with that method.

Case studies and presentations

Case studies and case presentations can be a good source of learning and an excellent way of improving both knowledge and practical skill. A case presentation is often a real case that one clinician presents to others, whilst a case study is usually a scenario or composite set of real or simulated conditions. Practice meetings can be a good time for case studies or case presentations. Used in this way, they can also be good presentation practice while skills such as communication, information transfer, clear presentation of material and responding to questions mean they are also a good source of experience/training for these 'soft' skills.

If the case is a real one then it must be anonymised and patient confidentiality maintained, unless the case is part of a professional team discussion with the purpose of providing care and treatment for a specific patient. While noted here, this use of case study is not a CPD activity.

Both can be used face to face with colleagues and underpin professional discussion and dialogue or they can be worked on individually, perhaps online or in a journal format. The latter format can be constructed within a verifiable CPD framework more easily than the former. However, it is the rich discussion with colleagues that makes this activity an excellent learning experience. The individual making the presentation may find it helpful to pose questions to those sharing the presentation, particularly where more than one option of care or treatment was available. This helps to enhance the learning for everyone present. Many case studies/ presentations are made to a multiprofessional group, including all members of the dental team, which broadens the learning experience and can also support good team working and cohesion.

Indemnity providers are often a rich source of case material across a wide range of topics, either on their websites or in their publications.

Clinical audit

> 'As a quality improvement mechanism audit can demonstrate that genuine and substantial efforts are being made by staff to deliver high-quality professional care to all their patients.'

(Scrivener *et al.*, 2002)

Few dental professionals can be unaware of audit. However, in my experience audit may not be used as effectively as it could be. As a tool, it can be employed in most aspects of dentistry. Audit provides evidence of improvements embedded within day-to-day practice. Over time, audit also evidences continuous improvement. Clinical audit is an activity that all UK dentists must undertake. In Scotland, it is part of the NHS terms of service and in England the CQC will want to see evidence of audits carried out (see below). NHS England can also request to see evidence of audit.

Clinical audit is part of clinical governance and quality improvement and as such, a record of the audit must be kept. This will include the audit outline, results and the changes made as a result of the findings (Figure 9.2).

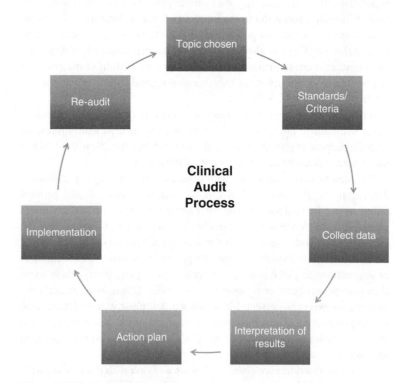

Figure 9.2 The clinical audit process.

Audit is a spiral activity, by which I mean not a 'one-off' event. It would be unusual for an initial, baseline audit to fully meet the standards set. Audits should be repeated to review how improvements have been implemented, ideally with each subsequent audit demonstrating higher standards and greater consistency than the one before. The key word with any audit is *improvement*.

The CQC in England requires dental practices to undertake three audits on the following topics (2017).

- *Infection prevention and control*: establish and operate a quality assurance system that covers the use of effective measures of decontamination and infection control. Complying with HTM01-05 (Decontamination in primary care dental practices) shows there are valid quality assurance systems in place. As a minimum, practices should audit their decontamination processes every 6 months, with an appropriate review dependent on audit outcomes. The Infection Prevention Society audit tool could be used.

- *X-rays*: current regulations for using ionising radiation for medical and dental purposes (both IRR99 and IR(ME)R2000) place a legal responsibility to establish and maintain quality assurance programmes for dental radiology. The consistent quality of radiographs must be assured through audit. There is an example audit under 'selection criteria for dental radiography 9.2.1' on the Faculty of General Dental Practice (FGDP) Standards in Dentistry online.

- *Accessibility*: all organisations providing services to the public must audit their facilities and ensure they comply with the Equality Act 2010.

There are a number of useful guides and publications about how to undertake audit with templates, for example, *The Clinical Audit and Peer Review Cookbook* (Wales Dental Deanery, 2015).

There are certain audit topics that are frequently found within GDC determinations. These include:

- record keeping
- radiographs
- periodontal examination and treatment
- antimicrobial prescribing.

As noted above, to undertake an audit the standard against which practice will be measured needs to be set. A good place to start is the standards and guidelines set by specialist societies and Royal Colleges. These are often the standards used by the GDC expert witnesses when reporting on evidence provided to a Practice Committee. The Faculty of General Practice (2007, 2013, 2014, 2016) publishes open access online standards and I recommend these as a good place to begin.

All audits should have a project outline including:
- aims and objectives
- summary of the methodology
- timetable
- detail of educational source material.

The Avon Primary Care Research Collaborative has some excellent resources for audit with a toolkit and templates: www.apcrc.nhs.uk.

Staff meetings

Staff meetings are essential for good team working and good business working of the practice, generally taking place every 1–2 months. Meetings should be no longer than an hour which means they need to be chaired well. A chair ensures that everyone keeps on topic and does not hog the meeting with their own agenda. While a staff meeting will not constitute CPD, the notes of staff meetings can be valuable evidence to meet GDC requirements as part of a determination in fitness to practise cases. If written well, they can show how a registrant has implemented new ways of working within the practice and demonstrate presentation of audit results, project working and engagement with colleagues. To be good evidence, the meeting needs to be documented properly. The headings you can consider when planning a meeting or writing up the staff meeting notes afterwards can include the following.
- Date and time of the meeting
- Who was present
- Apologies
- Review of actions from last meeting – what has been completed
- The topics discussed – key points from the discussion
- Action points – who will do what, by when?
- Date of next meeting

Patient surveys (feedback)

Patients are the life blood of dental practice so their satisfaction with the service and care provided is essential. Unlike general medical practitioners, whose patients are largely allocated to a practice, individuals choose their dental practice and dental professionals. If they do not like either the practice or the people who work there, they will move on. Patient loyalty is therefore extremely important to dentistry. Patient satisfaction is crucial and definitely worth checking and constantly keeping in touch with. A patient who is satisfied will tell others that they attend a good practice but a patient who is not satisfied is likely to tell far more people. Patient satisfaction affects the bottom line from a business point of view so dental professionals need to think seriously about monitoring patient satisfaction.

The NHS Management Inquiry (1983) pushed forward the use of patient satisfaction with its call for the collation of user opinion. Since then, patient satisfaction information has been gathered using a number of different formats, and electronic and hand-held technology has made it much easier to ask patients for their opinion. However, the questions themselves need to be carefully thought through if the response is to be of value.

Newsome and Wright (1999) reviewed the concept of patient satisfaction in their paper and found it to be 'a complex process balancing consumer expectations with perceptions of the service or product in question'.

Surveys and questionnaires are a good way of checking patient satisfaction, but the questions need to be carefully crafted if the responses are to be meaningful and not just tick box exercises. Some practices use telephone surveys to gain an understanding of how their patients feel about the practice. Others might use email to a group of patients, or an online survey method; others have patient forums. Whichever method is chosen, good questions are more likely to give good-quality information.

Parasuraman and Berry (1988) suggest considering the following characteristics when constructing a satisfaction questionnaire.

- *Reliability*: ability to perform the promised service dependably and accurately
- *Responsiveness*: willingness to help customers and provide prompt service
- *Assurance*: employees' knowledge and courtesy and their ability to inspire trust and confidence
- *Empathy*: caring, individualised attention given to customers
- *Tangibles*: appearance of physical facilities, equipment, personnel and written materials

These factors can be used to construct a patient questionnaire that provides good-quality useful feedback on both the overall practice and individual members of staff.

Zelthaml *et al.* (1990) suggest that:

> 'Service users who cannot judge the technical quality of the outcome effectively will base their quality judgements on structure and process dimensions such as physical settings, the ability to solve problems, to empathise, time-keeping, courtesy and so on.'

This work is particularly relevant to dentistry which has a high level of technical input. The patient will rarely be able to judge the quality of the dental procedure undertaken, but they will be able to judge whether the waiting area is comfortable and well furnished, whether the staff are polite, courteous and respectful and how long they are kept waiting. Patients can judge on many professional and behavioural characteristics of their dental team and this type of feedback is extremely useful and particularly so for a professional facing a challenge to their fitness to practise.

A sample questionnaire on the level of patient engagement is given at Appendix B. These type of questions can give useful data if the professional who is struggling has issues about communication, gaining informed consent or engaging with patients.

360° multisource feedback

360° feedback is part of multisource feedback and is a very useful tool to gauge a dental professional's understanding of their development needs. The essence of 360° feedback is that colleagues are asked to complete an anonymous questionnaire rating the individual and adding free text comments to assist them in improving their performance. It is important that the raters chosen fully understand that the objective is to give constructive, clear feedback to help the person being rated. This is not an opportunity to bring up old grudges or issues. Being critical is permissible, but not in a destructive manner.

To get a really good 360° picture, about 8–10 raters should be chosen; four or fewer is insufficient and the result is prone to bias. The raters should be a mix and include peers at the same level as the person being rated, individuals who may be line managed by the person or junior to them, and people who are senior. In the case of a dentist, that would be other dentists in the practice, dental nurses, practice managers, the principal or senior dentists, hygienists, therapists and receptionists. Finding the right number can be a challenge for a small practice or department. Colleagues from outside the practice can be asked to rate, but they do need to know the person quite well.

When raters have been selected, they will receive a series of questions and will rate those questions on a scale of usually 1–6, 6 being the best ever and 1 meaning the person has some serious development needs. Where the extremes of the scoring are used, people are encouraged to make comments on what could be improved or maintained. The individual undertaking the 360° completes the same questionnaire and rates themselves. The scores from all the raters are collated and the range analysed.

There are a number of online 360° tools and some paper tools as well. Be wary of those that do not have a human element for the feedback; the person being rated should not receive their results cold – they need to be interpreted.

The 360° is best run from outside the practice by someone independent. This increases the anonymity of the exercise and encourages people to be objective and honest in their feedback. This external person or company will collate the responses, make a report and feed back to the person being rated (in a positive, supportive way). The purpose is to help the person understand where they are better than they thought and where the areas for improvement are. It can be a scary exercise. The really interesting aspects of 360° are where the scores of the individual and the raters differ. These are the areas that are helpful to work on.

I have included a sample 360° feedback questionnaire at Appendix C. This has been specifically constructed to help with feedback on influencing skills.

Standards, national guidelines

Dental professionals are surrounded by a multitude of standards and national guidelines. In one sense this is good, but it can also be overwhelming. Standards and national guidelines can be excellent learning material, and are extremely useful when constructing a portfolio of evidence to present at a fitness to practise panel hearing. The GDC *Standards for the Dental Team* (2013) are the standards that all dental professionals are judged against; there are nine principles that are essentially ethical principles that must be followed. In addition, the GDC produces guidance on a number of issues. All dental professionals should be familiar with this.

- Guidance on advertising
- Guidance on child protection and vulnerable adults
- Guidance on commissioning and manufacturing dental appliances
- Guidance on indemnity
- Guidance on prescribing medicines
- Guidance on reporting criminal proceedings
- Guidance on using social media

Specialist dental societies and associations also produce helpful guidance and standards of working. In particular, clinical dental professionals should be familiar with those of the Faculty of General Dental Practice (UK) (www.fgdp.org.uk):

- Clinical Examination and Record Keeping
- Selection Criteria for Dental Radiography
- Antimicrobial Prescribing for GDPs.

In addition, the FGDP produces online learning materials that are very accessible:

- Standards in Dentistry
- Key Skills in Primary Dental Care
- Pathways in Practice.

Working with a mentor

'The process whereby an experienced, highly regarded, empathic person (the mentor) guides another individual (the mentee) in the development and re-examination of their own ideas, learning and personal and

professional development. The mentor who often, but not necessarily, works in the same organization or field as the mentee, achieves this by listening and talking in confidence to the mentee.'

(SCOPME, 1998)

A mentor has experience in the same profession/field as the mentee. Mentoring is not typically a relationship of equals; the mentor must have skill and expertise that the mentee requires and is seeking. When looking for a mentor, there are some things to consider.

- Experience in the career aspect in which you are interested.
- Someone with wide personal networks.
- Someone you respect and trust.
- Someone who has been trained in the role of mentor (they have mentoring skills as well as professional expertise).
- Someone motivational.
- Someone who is open and willing to share their own successes and failures.

A mentor should challenge the thinking of their mentee, especially if they are stuck on one perspective. Mentors can offer advice and ideas and the perceptive mentor will notice shifts in their mentee's thinking, identify new perspectives opening up and offer new understanding of what is possible. A mentor will be able to offer fresh insights, perhaps because they have dealt with similar situations in the past.

Working with a coach

'The coach works with clients to achieve speedy, increased and sustained effectiveness in their lives and careers through focused learning. The coach's sole aim is to work with the client to achieve all of the client's potential – as defined by the client.'

(Rogers, 2004)

A coach's attitude to their client/coachee is non-judgemental, caring and supportive of their situation and needs. They create an empathic environment so that the person being coached feels safe to discuss the issues that are of importance to them. The coaching conversation is a confidential one and dental professionals undertaking coaching can expect the same degree of confidentiality that they provide for their own patients.

Coaches help individuals achieve their goals. They do this by asking questions that identify the gap between what the person intends to do and what they are actually doing. A coach holds their coachee responsible for taking their own actions, doing the work necessary to achieve their goals and finding focus. The coach can 'hold a mirror' to reflect and understand the impact the coachee has on others. Coaching is supportive but not soft. Coaching challenges you to dig deep within yourself to reflect on how you behave and what your aspirations really are. Sometimes this can feel uncomfortable as you begin to understand yourself better and what motivates you.

A coach will ask relevant, probing questions, at times in challenging ways. Coaching conversations are not friendly chats; they have purpose and the coach provides focus, bringing the individual back to the intended outcomes of the conversation. A great coach does not have to be a dental professional, but they do need to have an understanding of the environment in which you work. However, the skills of coaching are different from the skills of being a dental professional and often it can be a bonus that they are not a dental professional as they can bring fresh insights to the issues.

You may be wondering what the difference is between coaching and mentoring. Both interventions use similar skills of listening, using focused questioning, reflecting back, paraphrasing and probing. The essential difference is that the mentor shares the same professional background as the person they are mentoring. The coach can but does not have to and often it is better if they are from a different background. Mentors share external expertise and advice, coaches help to uncover the expertise from within their coachee. A coach knows how to ask great questions to draw out insights, understanding and learning; a mentor knows how to answer great questions and pass on their experience, skill and expertise.

When considering who to ask to be either your mentor or your coach, ensure they have undertaken training and ideally have a qualification in mentoring or coaching or both. There are many excellent mentors and coaches who have 'learnt on the job', but times are moving on and having formal training ensures their skills have been honed.

Appendix A Personal development plan template

Name			
Date Plan Written		Date Plan Reviewed	
GDC domains			
Strengths			
Management & Leadership	Communication	Management & Leadership	Communication
Knowledge & Skill	Professional	Knowledge & Skill	Professional
		Weaknesses	
SHORT-TERM OBJECTIVES (up to 12 months)		LONG-TERM OBJECTIVES (12 – 24 months)	

Development Need Specfic	Activity chosen and method Achievable	Date Timed	Outcome expected	How outcome measured Measurable	How will this benefit patients? Relevant

Methods that you can use for your personal development

- Face to face courses
- On-line courses
- Audit
- Peer Review
- Case Based Discussion
- Working with a mentor
- Working with a coach
- Undertaking a project
- Shadowing
- Reflective log

A mixture of methods is best for all round development.

Appendix B   Patient engagement questionnaire

Here at Blankshire dental practice we are keen to improve our service to all our patients. We are particularly interested to ensure you feel fully involved in the dental care and treatment you receive. Please take a few minutes of your time to answer the questions below.

	Questions	Please circle the answer that is right for you
1	At your appointment today, were different treatment options discussed with you?	Yes No Not applicable
2	Did you understand the options that were discussed with you?	Yes No Not applicable
3	If you didn't understand the options at first, did the dentist help you to understand by explaining more or showing you an example?	Yes No Not applicable
4	Did the dentist listen to you?	Yes No
5	Do you feel the dentist spent enough time with you?	Yes No
6	Was the dentist polite?	Yes No
7	Were you able to ask all the questions you wanted to?	Yes No
8	Did you feel comfortable asking the questions you wanted to?	Yes No
9	Did the dentist speak clearly with words you were able to understand, not dental speak?	Yes No
10	Before your treatment started today, did the dentist explain what they were going to do?	Yes No

If you have any comments that you would like to make to help us improve what we do, please add them in the box below.

Thank you for taking the time to complete this questionnaire, your opinion is very important to us.

Please place your completed questionnaire in the box on the reception desk.

Appendix C   Influencing skills questionnaire – 360° colleague feedback

Thank you for taking the time to support your colleague by your honest and constructive feedback.

It is very important to personal development to understand how our colleagues view us. Please remember your colleague needs your feedback to be totally honest so they can work on maintaining their strengths and improving any weaknesses.

Your feedback and comments are totally anonymous and you will not be identified. Your colleague will have no knowledge of individuals nor the comments they make.

In the box to the right of each statement, write the number that best represents how often your colleague demonstrates that behaviour.

1 = Never 2 = Rarely 3 = Sometimes 4 = Often 5 = Very often 6 = Always
Name of person you are rating: ....

	Statement	Rating
1	Actively seeks feedback from others and uses this feedback to improve own practice and personal integrity	
2	Demonstrates a good knowledge of the regulations and standards relating to clinical practice	
3	Is aware of own competences and works within scope of practice	
4	Maintains clear and accurate records and understands the underpinning principles	
5	Can provide advice and support if asked by colleagues and can receive feedback from colleagues in the patient's best interest	
6	Contributes to the development of a robust clinical governance framework	
7	Consistently ensures patients are treated with dignity and respect	
8	Talks and listens to patients to improve services and resolve conflicts or dissatisfaction	
9	Can negotiate and resolve conflict in a positive manner	
10	Communicates effectively with patients/carers, ensuring they have understood information about their treatment and care	
11	Communicates in a manner appropriate for each individual	
12	Is fair and consistent in their approach	
13	Delegates appropriately, ensuring colleagues have the skill to carry out the task	
14	Listens to others' ideas, expertise and contributions to develop patient care and services	
15	Understands how own emotions, stress and prejudices can affect behaviour and judgement	
16	Understands how own role and responsibilities work within the dental team	
17	Accepts responsibility for own actions and omissions	

	Statement	Rating
18	Understands the importance of ethical decisions and values	
19	Consistently works in an open, honest and ethical manner	
20	Empowers others, within their scope of practice	
21	Contributes to problem solving, team building and adding improvements to service	
22	Establishes and maintains positive working relationships with others	
23	Maintains own professional skills through training and education, understanding the value of continuing professional development	
24	Understands the importance of raising concerns to protect patients	
25	Gets support from others by involving them in the decision-making process	
26	Shows people how their work is important to the broader goals of the practice	
27	Appeals to values or principles, such as concern for the patient, quality or fairness	
28	Looks for solutions that will benefit all parties involved	
29	Lets people know the negative consequences if they do not follow their wishes	
30	Takes time to understand other people's viewpoints and concerns	

Please use the box below to add your thoughts and suggestions for strengths and weaknesses that XXXX demonstrates and how they might work to develop and improve.

Narrative is very important and is particularly helpful if there are statements you have rated as either 1/2 (rarely or never) and 6 (always).

Please email your completed questionnaire to: by: (date)

References

Care Quality Commission (2017) *Audits in Primary Care Dental Services*. Available at: www.cqc.org.uk/guidance-providers/dentists/dental-mythbuster-17-audits-primary-care-dental-services (accessed 11 January 2018).

Chisholm, A., Shipway, J. and Tong, R. (2012) *Evaluation of Supporting Evidence Types for Revalidation, Stage 1*. Available at: file:///C:/Users/Owner/Downloads/ Evaluation%20of%20Supporting%20Evidence%20November%202012%20(Picker-GDC)%20Report.pdf (accessed 11 January 2018).

Clegg, S. and Bradley, S. (2006) Models of personal development: practices and processes. *British Educational Research Journal*, **32**(1), 57–76.

Faculty of General Dental Practice (UK) (2007) *Standards in Dentistry*. Available at: www.fgdp.org.uk.

Faculty of General Dental Practice (UK) (2013) *Selection Criteria for Dental Radiographs*. Available at: www.fgdp.org.uk.

Faculty of General Dental Practice (UK) (2014) *Antimicrobial Prescribing for General Dental Practitioners*. Available at: www.fgdp.org.uk.

Faculty of General Dental Practice (UK) (2016) *Clinical Examination and Record Keeping*. Available at: www.fgdp.org.uk.

General Dental Council (2013) *Standards for the Dental Team*. General Dental Council, London.

Healthcare Foundation (2012) *Pathway Peer Review to Improve Quality*. Available at: info@health.org.uk

Newsome, P.R.H. and Wright, G.H. (1999) Patient management: a review of patient satisfaction: 2. Dental patient satisfaction: an appraisal of recent literature. *British Dental Journal*, **186**, 166–170.

NHS Management Inquiry (1983) Department of Health and Social Security, London.

Parasuraman, A. and Berry, L. (1988) SERVQUAL: a multiple item scale for measuring consumer perceptions of service quality. *Journal of Retailing*, **64**, 12–40.

Rogers, J. (2004) *Coaching Skills: A Handbook*. Open University Press, Maidenhead.

Scrivener, R., Morrell, C., Baker, R. *et al.* (2002) *Principles for Best Practice in Clinical Audit*. Radcliffe Medical Press, Oxford.

Standing Committee on Postgraduate Medical and Dental Education (SCOPME) (1998) *Supporting Doctors and Dentists at Work. An Enquiry into Mentoring*. Standing Committee on Postgraduate Medical and Dental Education, London.

Wales Dental Deanery (2015) *Clinical Audit and Peer Review Cookbook*, Version 2. Available at https://dental.walesdeanery.org/sites/default/files/1b._the_cookbook_-_a_ guide_to_undertaking_a_clinical_audit_0.pdf (accessed 11 January 2018).

Zelthaml, V., Parasuraman, A. and Berry, L. (1990) *Delivering Quality Service*. Free Press, New York.

Chapter 10 **Supporting colleagues who struggle**

In this final chapter I will cover the skills needed to support a colleague who is struggling with their performance. First I will discuss the personal attributes that a good supporter should cultivate to become a great supporter. Then I will look at reflective practice and some of the models that a supporter can introduce to encourage reflective skills. These are essential for someone who is struggling with performance concerns. Finally, I will cover a number of tools that work well when used in a 1:1 situation. Many of the tools covered in Chapter 9 will also be of help. Chapter 8 looked at insight and self-awareness which are also particularly relevant for supporters.

To begin, I want to think about the personal skills that are needed when supporting a colleague. These include:

- being non-judgemental
- listening
- paraphrasing
- questioning
- guiding

Being non-judgemental

When supporting a colleague who is struggling or for whom there is a cause for concern, it is important not to judge them. Any dental professional can struggle at any time in their career and the reasons and underpinning factors are many and complex. A great supporter does not bring judgement to the table.

Listening

Really listening to another person is not easy. It's often called 'active listening'. You would think that dental professionals would be good at listening. However, when a supporter is listening, they are not thinking about what to say in response, or wondering if they switched off the lights at home or what to have for tea – they are really listening to their colleague. They listen to the

---

How to Survive Dental Performance Difficulties, First Edition. Janine Brooks.
© 2018 John Wiley & Sons Ltd. Published 2018 by John Wiley & Sons Ltd.

words and the spaces between words, the emotions, feelings and values being expressed. They are watching for the non-verbal cues and signs.

Paraphrasing

There is a real skill in being able to reflect back to the person what you have heard and sensed. Good reflecting creates rapport and trust between the supporter and their colleague. The ability to reflect accurately can help to clarify issues for the individual. A skilful supporter will be able to reflect back not only the language and terminology they have heard, but also aspects of character, for example 'That took courage'. Reflecting back the space between the words and what hasn't been said is also important.

Questioning

Asking the right questions at the right time, in the right way, is important to the supportive conversation. Phrasing questions is a skill, as is the way they are asked. It's usually best to avoid questions beginning with 'Why?' as they can make the individual feel defensive or as if they are being blamed. The tone of voice is also important to prevent the question being received as an accusation.

Guiding

This is a collection of all the skills above, plus the ability to bring enthusiasm, encouragement and analysis to the conversation. This is often where the supporter can bring their experience and advice, suggest resources the individual can try, relate their own experiences and offer opinions. I sometimes think of this skill as signposting, helping another find their way and seek out the resources they need to get back on track.

Reflective practice/writing and learning

Helping a colleague learn to use reflection well and confidently is a great gift. Once learned, it reaps rewards many times over.

> *'If you keep on doing what you've always done, you'll keep on getting what you've always got.'*

> (author unknown)

This quote is so true. Often when an error has occurred, insufficient time and thought are given to why it occurred. Even if the why and the how are known, if changes are not made then the error is likely to happen again and again.

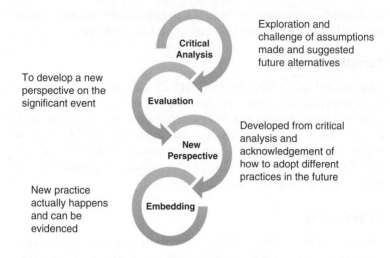

Figure 10.1 What's involved in reflection?

Reflective practice is a way of taking stock of what has happened, making sense of the experience and taking the learning forward (Figure 10.1). It is a structured process of noticing and evaluation. Reflection enables learning. It makes it easier to break the cycle of doing what you've always done. The good news is that most of us do it, although not always consciously.

The roots of reflective practice
Some authors believe that reflective learning is as important as knowledge derived from empirical research (Joyce-McCoach and Smith, 2016). It seems reasonable that the day-to-day experience gained from undertaking activities is as important as research conducted under controlled conditions. It's not an either/or, both are needed.

The roots of reflective practice probably begin with Dewey (1859–1952), an American pragmatist philosopher who considered thinking to be a form of experimentation, a way of doing. Central to Dewey's approach to education was learning from experience, by doing and then reflecting on what happened. Dewey and Schön advocated on-the-spot reflection in real time (not looking back). Donald Schön (1983) made the differentiation between reflection as the action is happening – reflection *in* action – and reflection after the event – reflection *on* action. The latter includes review, analysis and evaluation of the situation. In dentistry, an example of reflection in action would be clinicians reflecting as they cut cavities, crown or implant preparations whether the operation is progressing as it should and making small changes as they go along.

There are many ways of being reflective and undertaking reflective practice. It is a practice-based discipline, but it must be underpinned by theory.

Johns (2004) views reflection as a form of introspection (self-transformation). Interestingly, he suggests reflection is *not* primarily a technology to produce better patient outcomes, but is essentially about personal growth.

Guided reflection cannot be done alone. It is profoundly difficult for practitioners to see beyond themselves, to their own self-distortions and limited horizons. This can fit with coaching and mentoring where the individual works face to face with a skilled supporter, coach or mentor and is guided in their reflection by an expert.

'Maybe reflective practices offer us a way of trying to make sense of the uncertainty in our workplaces and the courage to work competently and ethically at the edge of order and chaos ...'

(Ghaye, 2000, p. 7)

This quote is taken from the first edition of the *Journal of Reflective Practice*. Tony Ghaye wrote the editorial 'Into the effective mode: bridging the stagnant moat'. The quote strikes a chord for me and seems particularly pertinent to dentistry and dental practice.

'Engaging in regular reflection enables practitioners to manage the personal and professional impact of addressing their patients' fundamental health and wellbeing needs on a daily basis.'

(Oelofsen, 2012)

Oelofsen, a consultant clinical psychologist, writes here about using reflective practice and learning in the field of nursing. The message works for all healthcare professionals.

Reflective practice is a fundamental part of lifelong learning. The General Dental Council Standards for the Dental Team include as Standard 7: *Maintain, develop and work within your professional knowledge and skill* (GDC, 2013). Specifically, your CPD activity should improve your practice. Reflective practice is key to taking the learning from an educational activity and translating it into action and improved practice. To reflect in a meaningful way means the dental professional needs to examine their assumptions about their everyday work. To do that, professionals must have self-awareness and be able to critically evaluate their own reactions to their environment. Reflective practice and writing is a helpful activity to enhance insight and can underpin the work outlined in Chapter 8.

Reflective models

There are a number of models that can help individuals to reflect methodically. They can be particularly helpful when first using reflection. Here I will cover one model, Gibbs, in some detail. Other models are included in the references at the end of the chapter.

When something doesn't go to plan, it is helpful to unpick the reasons why. If we don't understand why something didn't work, it is hard to do something differently next time. There is also a danger that the errors and mistakes are repeated time and again.

Gibbs model (1998)

Gibbs originally developed his cycle as a way of debriefing following an event or experience (Figure 10.2). Initially adopted by nursing, it has spread throughout healthcare as a way to aid reflection. Gibbs' model brings together

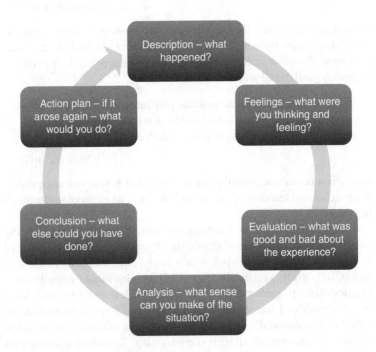

Figure 10.2 Gibbs reflective model.

theory and experience and these two go hand in hand, complementing each other around the cycle. Gibbs' is a good model to kickstart reflective learning. It helps the individual to think systematically through all the phases of an experience.

I will expand a little more on the stages of this model.

- *Description*: this is setting the scene and the context of the experience chosen to reflect upon. Try to keep the information here relevant and not excessive.
- *Feelings*: here the individual needs to think about the feelings and emotions they experienced during the situation they are reflecting upon. Self-awareness is key in thinking through the impact the experience had on the individual and others involved.
- *Evaluation*: this is where the person thinks about how well they think things went. Relevant theory and underpinning knowledge could also be included here. Think about whether judgements were good or flawed.
- *Analysis*: at this point in the reflection, include what helped and what got in the way of success. The experience could be compared with underpinning knowledge. Break down the event and analyse each part separately, which will enhance the learning.
- *Conclusion*: here the person thinks about whether they could have done anything differently. What have they learned from the experience and how could they replicate a good experience to increase their success in the future?
- *Action plan*: finally, this step makes the individual commit to what they will do differently and what they intend to change.

Writing reflectively

Whilst writing a reflection can help it to be more robust and meaningful, most dental professionals do not write their reflections down. However, if there is a fitness to practise case or where reflections are part of enhanced CPD, written reflections will be required. Writing in a reflective way is not easy to do, certainly not at first. We are used to writing description, not reflection. It can take a little while to get it right. To help, I have included examples of the same scenario but written in three different ways so that the difference is more obvious.

The following three accounts are of a presentation at a practice team meeting by a 24-year-old Foundation trainee. The accounts are of the same event written at three different levels of reflection. Reviewing the accounts together should help to demonstrate what is description and what is reflection and, even more, what is deeper reflection that generates real learning.

(A)

I had to take an agenda item to the regular team meeting in my second month of working at High Town dental practice. I had to talk about the project that I am on (creating a new database for the reception information system). I had done a presentation before and then I relied on my acting skills. Despite the acting, I spent quite a bit of time preparing it in the way that I have seen others make similar presentations.

The presentation at the last team meeting, given by my colleague, went well; she used PowerPoint and I decided to use it. I decided that a good presentation comes from good planning and having all the figures that anyone might request so I spent a long time in the preparation and I went in feeling confident.

However, I became nervous when I realised they were all waiting for me to speak and my nerves made my voice wobble. I did not know how to stop it. Early on, I noticed that people seemed not to understand what I was saying despite the PowerPoint. Using PowerPoint meant that people received my presentation both through what I was saying and what I had prepared on the slides. In a way that meant they got it twice but I noticed that Mrs Shaw (my trainer) repeated bits of what I had said several times and once or twice answered questions for me. This made me feel uncomfortable. I felt it was quite patronising and I was upset. Later, my colleagues said that she always does it. I was disappointed that my presentation did not seem to have gone well.

I thought about the presentation for several days and then talked with Mrs Shaw about the presentation (there was no one else). She gave me a list of points for improvement next time. They included putting less on PowerPoint, talking more slowly and calming myself down in some way.

I also have to write down the figures in a different way so that they can be understood better. She suggested that I should do a presentation to several of the team sometime next week so that I can improve my performance.

(B)

I had to take an agenda item to the regular team meeting in my second month of working at High Town dental practice. I had to talk about the project that I am on. I am creating a new database for the reception information system. I had given a presentation before and that time I relied on my acting skills. I did realise that there were considerable differences between then and now, particularly in the situation (it was only fellow students and my tutor before). I was confident but I did spend quite a bit of time preparing. Because everyone else here uses PowerPoint, I felt I had better use it – though I realised that it was not for the best reasons. I also prepared lots of figures so that I could answer questions. I thought, at that stage, that any questions would involve requests for data. When I think back on the preparation that I did, I realise that I was desperately trying to prove that I could make a presentation as well as my colleague, who did the last one. I wanted to impress everyone. I had not realised there was so much to learn about presenting, and how much I needed to know about PowerPoint to use it properly.

When I set up the presentation in the meeting I tried to be calm but it did not work out. Early on, the PowerPoint went wrong and I began to panic. Trying to pretend that I was cool and confident made the situation worse because I did not admit my difficulties and ask for help. The more I spoke, the more my voice went wobbly. I realised, from the kinds of questions that the others asked, that they did not understand what I was saying. They were asking for clarification – not the figures. I felt worse when Mrs Shaw, my trainer, started to answer questions for me. I felt flustered and even less able to cope.

As a result of this poor presentation, my self-esteem is low at work now. I had thought I was doing all right in the practice. After a few days, I went to see Mrs Shaw and we talked it over. I still feel that her interventions did not help me. Interestingly, several of my colleagues commented that she always does that. It was probably her behaviour, more than anything else, that damaged my poise. Partly through talking over the presentation and the things that went wrong (but not, of course, her interventions), I can see several areas that I could get better. I need to know more about using PowerPoint – and to practise with it. I recognise, also, that my old acting skills might have given me initial confidence, but I needed more than a clear voice, especially when I lost my way with PowerPoint. Relying on a mass of figures was not right either. It was not figures they wanted. In retrospect, I could have put the figures on a handout. I am hoping to have a chance to try with a presentation, practising with some of the team.

(C)

I am writing this back in at home. It all happened 2 days ago.

Two months after I started at High Town dental practice, I had to take an agenda item to the team meeting. I was required to report on my progress in the project on which I am working. I am developing a new database for the reception information system of the practice. I was immediately worried. I was scared about not saying the right things and not being able to answer questions properly. I did a presentation in my course at university and felt the same about it initially. I was thinking then, like this time, I could use my acting skills. Both times that was helpful in maintaining my confidence at first, at least. Though the fact that I was all right last time through the whole presentation may not have helped me this time!

I decided to use PowerPoint. I was not very easy about its use because I have seen it go wrong so often. However, I have not seen anyone else give a presentation here without using it – and learning to use PowerPoint would be valuable. I was not sure, when it came to the session, whether I really knew enough about running PowerPoint. (How do you know when you know enough about something? Dummy runs, I suppose, but I couldn't get the laptop when I wanted it.)

When it came to the presentation, I really wanted to do it well – as well as the presentations were done the meeting before. Maybe I wanted too much to do well. Previous presentations have been interesting, informative and clear and I thought the handouts from them were good (I noticed that the best gave enough but not too much information).

In the event, the session was a disaster and has left me feeling uncomfortable in my work and I even worry about it at home. I need to think about why a simple presentation could have such an effect on me. The PowerPoint went wrong (I think I clicked on the wrong thing). My efforts to be calm and 'cool' failed and my voice went wobbly – that was, anyway, how it felt to me. My colleague actually said afterwards that I looked quite calm despite what I was feeling (I am not sure whether she meant it or was trying to help me). When I think back to that moment, if I had thought that I still looked calm (despite what I felt), I could have regained the situation. As it was, it went from bad to worse and I know that my state became obvious because Mrs Shaw, my trainer, began to answer the questions that people were asking for me.

I am thinking about the awful presentation again – it was this time last week. I am reading what I wrote earlier about it. Now I return to it, I do have a slightly different perspective. I think that it was not as bad as it felt at the time. Several of my colleagues told me afterwards that Mrs Shaw always steps in to answer questions like that and they commented that I handled her intrusion well. That is interesting. I need to do some thinking about how to act next time to prevent this interruption from happening or to deal with the situation when she starts*. I might look in the library for that book on assertiveness.

I have talked to Mrs Shaw now too. I notice that my confidence in her is not all that great while I am still feeling a bit cross. However, I am feeling more positive generally and I can begin to analyse what I could do better in the presentation. It is interesting to see the change in my attitude after a week. I need to think from the beginning about the process of giving a good presentation. I am not sure how helpful was my reliance on my acting skills*. Acting helped my voice to be stronger and better paced, but I was not just trying to put over someone else's lines but my own and I needed to be able to discuss matters in greater depth rather than just give the line*.

I probably will use PowerPoint again. I have had a look in the manual and it suggests that you treat it as a tool – not let it dominate and not use it as a means of presenting myself. That is what I think I was doing. I need not only to know how to use it, but I need to feel sufficiently confident in its use so I can retrieve the situation when things go wrong. That means understanding more than just the sequence of actions*.

As I am writing this, I am noticing how useful it is to go back over things I have written about before. I seem to be able to see the situation differently. The first time I wrote this, I felt that the presentation was dreadful and that I could not have done it differently. Then later I realised that there were things I did not know at the time (e.g. about Mrs Shaw and her habit of interrupting). I also recognise some of the areas in which I went wrong. At the time, I could not see that. It was as if my low self-esteem got in the way. Knowing where I went wrong, and admitting the errors to myself gives me a chance to improve next time – and perhaps to help Mrs Shaw to improve in her behaviour towards us!

*I have asterisked the points that I need to address in order to improve.

Each of the accounts takes the same scenario as its subject, but they are clearly different in the way the scenario is considered. Table 10.1 highlights the differences between each account and points to the content which is reflective.

When writing reflectively it can be useful to follow the steps shown in Figure 10.3.

Sharing your reflection with a mentor or coach can be beneficial in deepening the learning and getting maximum benefit from the process. Figure 10.4 sums up what being reflective means for the individual.

Table 10.1 Comparative analysis of the three written accounts.

Account	Analysis
A	The account describes what happened, sometimes mentioning past experiences, sometimes anticipating the future – but all in the context of an account of the event.
	There are some references to the VT's emotional reactions, but they have not explored how the reactions relate to their behaviour.
	Ideas are taken on without questioning them or considering them in depth.
	The account is written only from the VT's point of view.
	External information is mentioned but its impact on behaviour is not subject to consideration.
	Generally, one point is made at a time and ideas are not linked.
	This account is descriptive and contains little reflection
B	There is description of the event, but where there are external ideas or information,the material is subjected to consideration and deliberation.
	The account shows some analysis.
	There is recognition of the worth of exploring motives for behaviour.
	There is willingness to be critical of action.
	Relevant and helpful detail is explored where it has value.
	There is recognition of the overall effect of the event on self – in other words, there is some 'standing back' from the event.
	The account is written at one point in time. It does not, therefore, demonstrate the recognition that views can change with time and more reflection. In other words, the account does not indicate a recognition that frames of reference affect the manner in which we reflect at a given time.
	An account showing evidence of some reflection
C	Self-questioning is evident (an 'internal dialogue' is set up at times) deliberating between different views of her own behaviour (different views of her own and others).
	The VT takes into account the views and motives of others and considers these against her own.
	The VT recognises how prior experience and thoughts (own and others') interact with the production of her own behaviour.
	There is clear evidence of standing back from an event.
	The VT helps herself to learn from the experience by splitting off the reflective processes from the points she wants to learn (by asterisk system).
	There is recognition that the personal frame of reference can change according to the emotional state in which it is written, the acquisition of new information, the review of ideas and the effect of time passing.
	This account shows quite deep reflection, and it does incorporate a recognition that the frame of reference with which an event is viewed can change

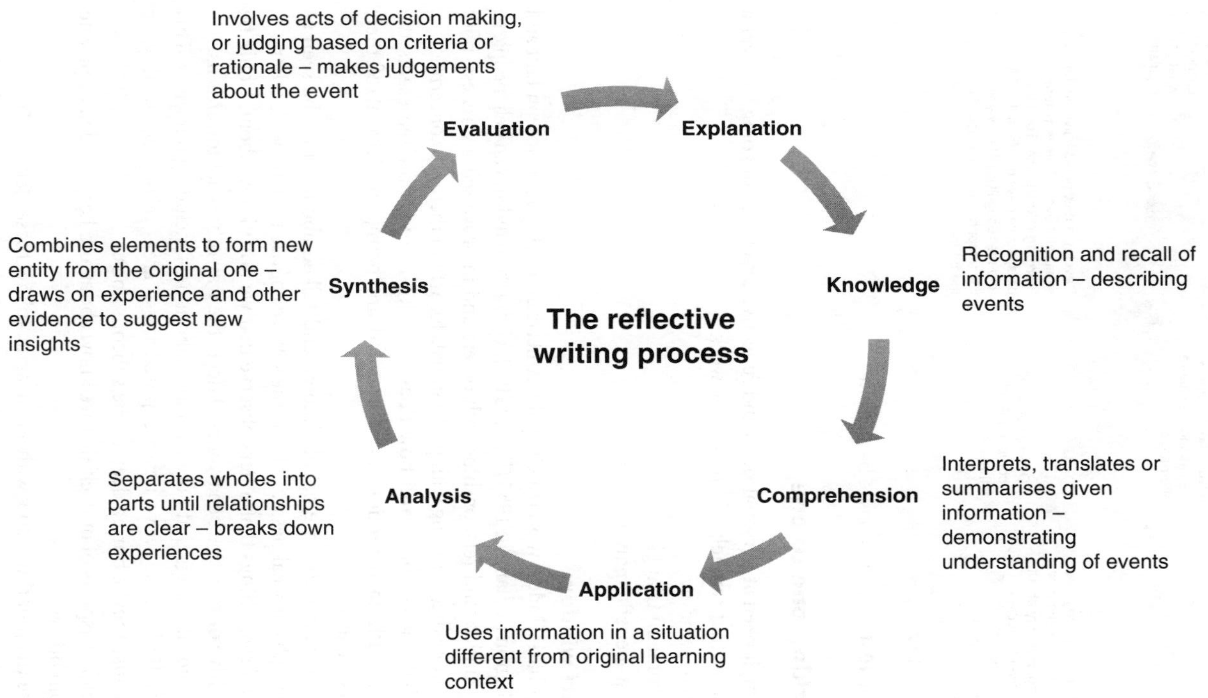

Recognition and recall of information – describing events

Interprets, translates or summarises given information – demonstrating understanding of events

Uses information in a situation different from original learning context

Separates wholes into parts until relationships are clear – breaks down experiences

Combines elements to form new entity from the original one – draws on experience and other evidence to suggest new insights

Involves acts of decision making, or judging based on criteria or rationale – makes judgements about the event

Knowledge

Comprehension

Application

Analysis

Synthesis

Evaluation

Explanation

The reflective writing process

Figure 10.3 The reflective writing process.

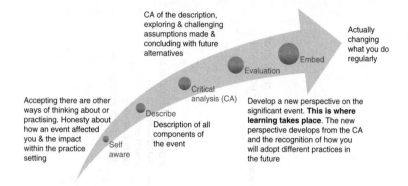

Figure 10.4 What it means to be reflective.

Working one to one

Having looked at personal skills and reflective practice, I'm going to cover a few tools that can help in one-to-one work.

- Johari window
- Karpmann triangle
- Cost–benefit analysis

Johari window

The Johari window was created by the American psychologists Joseph Luft and Harrington Ingham, in 1955 (Figure 10.5). Using the window can help people to better understand relationships with others and improve self-awareness, both important when working with professionals for whom there are concerns.

What does it mean and how does it work? The window represents the person with each section, pane or quadrant being an element of their self-awareness.

- *Open*: things that are openly known and talked about – may be seen as strengths or weaknesses. This is the self we choose to share with others.
- *Blind spot*: things that others observe that we don't know about. Could be positive or negative behaviours. Affects the way others act towards us.
- *Unknown*: things that nobody knows about us – including ourselves. This may be because we've never exposed those areas of our personality, or because they're buried deep in the subconscious.
- *Hidden*: aspects of our self that we know about and keep hidden or private from others.

To use the Johari window with a colleague, follow these steps.

- The person you are supporting draws the window; the panes can be different sizes to show how each section makes up the whole.
- Ask them to talk through each pane with you and explain why they have drawn the panes the size they have. For example, perhaps they have drawn

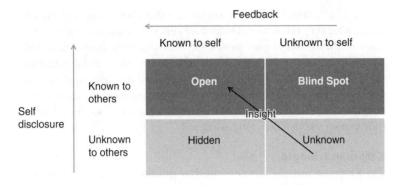

Figure 10.5 Johari window.

the open pane as the dominant area, much larger than the other three. Talking it through will help the person to reassess what they think about themselves. Encourage the individual to think about the differences in the size of the panes and why they think this is. The supporter can help the person think about the relationship between different panes and what that can tell them about themselves.

- Quadrant sizes can change over time with different circumstances.
- Feedback from others can increase the open quadrant and reduce the blind spot.
- When a person tells another things, the open quadrant increases and the hidden quadrant reduces.
- The supporter will help the individual to make a plan to change the relative size of the quadrants.

When to use insight
As with a number of tools that need facilitation, it's important to wait until the level of rapport between the supporter and the individual allows honest, open conversation. It can't be introduced at the first meeting. The Johari window can help the individual see themselves in relation to others around them. They can begin to ask if there is a mismatch between the way they view themselves and how others see them. As they work through the window with their supporter, they can reduce some of those mismatches. It may take time for some to share their thinking and feeling beyond the superficial and this will be affected by how they trust the relationship with their supporter.

Advantages and disadvantages
The advantages of the Johari window are that it helps raise self-awareness and also helps to review assumptions the person may have made about their life. By doing that, insight is improved.

The disadvantages of Johari's window are that some people tell the supporter what they think they should; they either don't take the exercise seriously or they use it to play games. Occasionally, some people may make inappropriate disclosures either about their private life or about patients or staff. The supporter will need to decide how confidentiality applies to the disclosure made and discuss that with the person they are working with before they start. Serious patient safety issues or concerns for the safety of a third person will definitely ring alarm bells.

Karpman triangle

The Karpman triangle was developed by psychiatrist Steven Karpman in 1968 (Figure 10.6). Karpman has undertaken work on transactional analysis and the triangle is a way of describing interactions between people. It can also be called the drama triangle or victim triangle. Using the triangle can help to unstick unhelpful patterns of behaviour, particularly if they are hidden or buried or not acknowledged by the person. Once uncovered, those unhelpful behaviours can be acknowledged and then they can be changed.

The triangle depicts three prime positions: the persecutor, the victim and the rescuer. At any one time, people can take on the behaviours and act out the role. The roles are linked and making changes to one will affect the other two.

- Persecutor – it's all your fault
- Victim – woe is me
- Rescuer – let me help you

When can it help?
Using the triangle with a skilled facilitator can help to raise awareness of patterns and habituated behaviours that can block and prevent change.

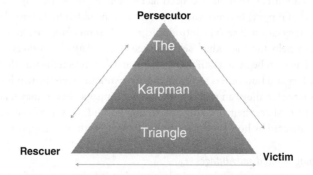

Figure 10.6 Karpman triangle.

How does it work?

The individual who is facing a complaint or a fitness to practise investigation may talk about feeling helpless (the victim) and look to someone else to solve their problem (the rescuer – coach/mentor or supporter). They may also see the person or organization who uncovered the cause for concern as the persecutor. This may also be the patient who made a complaint. When supporting a colleague who appears to be within the triangle, you can challenge the victim role and help them take control. Once they take back control, they can begin to see more clearly how to get themselves out of the difficulty.

Sometimes people can become stuck in one of the roles.

- *Stuck rescuer*: someone stuck in this role is always doing things for others. This can have the effect of disempowering staff and reducing team working. Helping them to realise that can help in more appropriate delegation and letting people do things for themselves.
- *Stuck persecutor*: some dental professionals may feel they have to constantly be in charge and always in control, which can lead others to see them as the persecutor.
- *Stuck victim*: some people can find a strange comfort in feeling that they are always the victim and that no matter how hard they try, they will always be a victim. This can lead to them not trying, because they tell themselves they will fail.

When supporting someone using the Karpman triangle, it is worth bearing in mind that for some people there are pay-offs for remaining in one particular role. Getting them to move out of that means they will have to be convinced that the pay-off for letting go is greater than that for remaining stuck.

Advantages and disadvantages

The advantages of using this technique are that people can find it liberating to think about the roles, where they see themselves and where they perceive others to be. It can increase self-awareness and encourage people to generate different strategies.

The disadvantages are that the model can be too challenging for those who are stuck in long-term patterns or with long-term conceptions of the role others play. There is also the issue of payback, as mentioned above.

Cost–benefit analysis

Cost–benefit analysis can be helpful in encouraging an individual to consider the costs of a particular action compared to its benefits. It can be useful when evaluating and re-evaluating goals and it can help those who are struggling to change what they are doing in ways that others expect of them, for example the benefits of undertaking a programme of remediation compared to the cost of not doing so. It is useful when supporting someone to think about costs and benefits of possible actions. The more detailed the factors that are to be analysed, the more robust will be the outcome.

Cost–benefit analysis can be used to test commitment or evaluate different options to move forward.

How does it work?

Support the person to clarify their goal, what they want for their future, what is important to them. Then ask them to list the potential advantages of achieving that goal, for themselves, the people around them and in the wider context of their life. Then ask them to list the disadvantages of achieving their goal. When that is done, an added refinement is to weight the advantages and disadvantages, which makes it a little easier to compare the two lists.

Advantages and disadvantages

The advantages of the technique are that it strengthens commitment and allows the individual to decide that the gain they will make is worth the effort. It is also useful for testing out how realistic a course of action actually is.

The disadvantage is that the person may discover that their goal is either not right or not realistic; this can seem like a failure and they may become disheartened. Should this occur, the support needs to be increased while they re-evaluate their goals.

Force field analysis

Force field analysis is a decision-making tool created in the 1940s by Kurt Lewin (1946, 1951), a social psychologist. It can be helpful when weighing the advantages or disadvantages of making a change and whether the proposed change is worth implementing. It helps in exploring and reviewing the factors (forces) that drive change and the forces that resist change. If change is to be successfully made, then the forces that drive the change must be stronger than the forces that resist or obstruct the change.

The aim of force field analysis is to understand all the forces that act upon the change or decision to be made. It can be used by an individual or a group.

How to use force field analysis

1. Describe the plan for change.
2. Identify the forces in favour of the change; include internal and external forces.
3. Identify the forces working against the change.
4. Assign scores to each force: 1 = weak, 5 = strong. Add up the totals.
5. Analyse and consider:

- whether to move forward or not
- how strong the forces are. Which are key? Can the forces be changed?
- whether you can strengthen the factors in favour of the change or reduce the obstructing forces.

When thinking about forces, include people (allies and opponents), attitudes, technology, equipment, ethical and legal factors, structures, etc.

Remember the following points.

- Force field analysis is a subjective tool and it is often best to use it as an adjunct to other tools, for example decision tree analysis or cost–benefit analysis.
- It takes time to add in as many factors as possible.
- Changing one force may impact on the others.

When drawing the diagram, weaker forces are often given a shorter or thinner line, stronger forces a longer/thicker line and moderate forces a medium line.

Advantages and disadvantages

The advantages of force field analysis are that you can visualise the forces and summarise them; it also allows the inclusion of qualitative factors and can help to highlight what can and cannot be changed.

The disadvantages are that a useful analysis needs full, accurate information. The technique is subjective and may oversimplify relationships between factors. In addition, it may increase conflict between those who are in favour of the change and those opposed to it.

How can supporters use force field analysis?

The supporter can help by explaining the tool and then supporting their colleague to think of all the factors that are relevant. In addition, they can test how strong the factors are. Finally, supporters can work with their colleague to increase their clarity about the factors impacting on the decision they wish to make. I've given an example of how force field analysis could be applied to dental practice in Figure 10.7.

Neurological levels

The work of Robert Dilts (1990) can help in understanding where an underpinning factor is located. Dilts developed the model of neurological levels, based on the work of Gregory Bateson (1972). The model describes a number of levels which can be used when supporting someone to make changes (Figure 10.8). The levels also help when looking at degrees of thinking. The model is closely aligned to NLP (see Chapter 8).

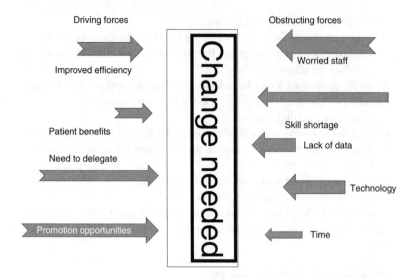

Figure 10.7 Practical application of force field analysis: introduce a new management structure into the practice.

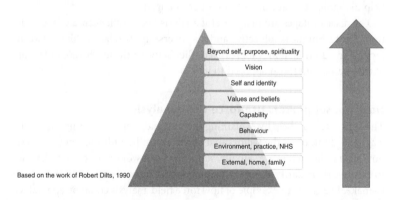

Figure 10.8 Neurological levels.

Using neurological levels, it is possible to target where help is needed and support should be applied. It is also possible to see how the levels interact. This will indicate how deeply embedded the issues are and affect the amount of change that is needed.

- *Beyond identity*: this is the 'for what?' or 'for whom?'. For some, that might be their religion or spirituality but it could also mean for the good of others. It is the way individuals make sense of why they do what they do.

- *Identity*: this is about who the person is and how they perceive themselves; essentially, how they fit into the big picture of life. It includes the role(s) they play and how they see their purpose. A dental professional might see themselves as a key player with responsibilities to other people (patients). Some individuals might perceive themselves to be very important while others might perceive themselves to be very unimportant. Behaviours, beliefs and values will interweave with identity.
- *Beliefs and values*: this is the 'why'. This is a person's fundamental core. Beliefs and values are what we use to make sense of what happens in our life. They underpin our capability and how we behave, what we consider to be important and what we do not. Beliefs and values are the map that individuals use when understanding what is important to them.
- *Capabilities*: this is how we are. Capabilities are our skill set. The clinical skills of a dental professional are part of this level.
- *Behaviour*: what a person does. Behaviour is the actions and reactions an individual exhibits.
- *Environment*: the 'where and when', the context in which we are. Environment is a broad level that includes the workplace (surgery, clinic), external surroundings, home, work patterns and much more.

Field and Field (2014) use the following sentence to demonstrate the different levels; the emphasis on the words changes depending on the neurological level.

I can't do that **here**	Environment
I can't do **that** here	Behaviour
I can't **do** that here	Capability
I **can't** do that here	Beliefs/values
I can't do that here	Identity

When supporting a dental professional who is struggling, it is helpful to think through their neurological levels with them to see if there are any keys that can help to motivate their remediation. When considering training plans to assist with remediation, capability alone is rarely sufficient; it must be teamed with behaviour and beliefs and values. Another use of neurological levels is to map the words that people use or the statements they make onto the levels, which can help to determine where they are coming from. Knowing that allows others (mentor or coach) to respond to them appropriately.

Examples of the areas that a supporter can explore and the sort of questions that will be relevant are given below (I have added Mission/Vision, which could be expressions of Beyond Identity).

- *Mission/vision*: where is the person going? What is central to their vision?
- *Identity*: self-esteem, job, home, self-worth; who you are.

- *Beliefs and values*: whether something is possible or impossible, what is the motivation, do the person's values and beliefs hinder or help them?
- *Capabilities*: what are the person's internal behaviours? How effectively do they use their skills?
- *Behaviour*: actions (what you do); include what an observer might see, hear or feel.
- *Environment*: surroundings, people and places the person interacts with. I have subdivided this into work and home.

The levels impact upon each other; the lower levels underpin the higher levels and vice versa. Improvements to the lower levels will be experienced at the higher levels. For example, if change is made in the environment, this can affect behaviour and capability or skill. If change is made at the capability/skill level, this can improve identity and enhance self-esteem and self-worth.

- *Identity*: I am a dental professional.
- *Beliefs and values*: oral health is important. People need good oral health.
- *Capabilities*: I am a skilled, experienced, conscientious clinician.
- *Behaviour*: I provide the best dentistry I can.
- *Environment*: my workplace operates a supportive, well-equipped, well-staffed practice.

When using neurological levels, it is important to listen to what the person you are supporting says, as this will help to locate their statement(s) somewhere on the levels. This helps to appreciate and understand where they are coming from.

Distinguishing between behaviour and identity.

This is an important distinction to make. Think about the following.

Ask someone 'What do you do?' (behaviour). If they answer 'I am ...' (identity) then they are equating behaviour and identity as the same. As an example, if you ask a dentist 'What do you do?' and they answer 'I am a dentist' then they are bringing Behaviour and Identity together into a single concept. This may not seem relevant or important until you consider what happens when a dentist stops doing what it is they do. Does this affect their perception of their identity? I suspect it does. Such a change can come about due to retirement or redundancy. However, it can also come about during fitness to practise proceedings. The individual may find their perception of their identity is under attack when their behaviour (and/or capability) is questioned. This was illustrated in case study 1 in Chapter 7.

Knowledge and use of neurological levels can be an important tool when making change; for example, knowing what an individual wants to achieve at all levels can increase motivation, identify and remove 'road blocks'. Changes often ripple down to the levels below, so a change in identity (the person's sense of who they are) can ripple down to beliefs and values, capabilities, behaviour and environment.

Conclusion

This chapter has covered a number of tools that supporters may find useful when working with colleagues for whom there are concerns. I hope that you have found the book helpful when considering the performance difficulties that dental professionals can find themselves in. I also hope that all dental professionals will find much in the book to assist them in building their personal toolkit of resources. I think there is something of value for every dental professional, no matter what stage you are in your career. Finally, for those who are currently struggling with fitness to practise issues, I sincerely hope the book will prove of use in not only surviving the difficulties but using the experience to 'return with the elixir'.

References

Bateson, G. (1972) *Steps to an Ecology of Mind*. University of Chicago Press, Chicago, IL.

Dilts, R. (1990) *Changing Belief Systems with Neuro Linguistic Programming*. Meta Publications, Capitola, CA.

Field, J. and Field, S. (2014) NLP Practitioner, Module 1. Available at: www.field-field.com.

General Dental Council (GDC) (2013) *Standards for the Dental Team*. General Dental Council, London.

Ghaye, T. (2000) Into the reflective mode: bridging the stagnant moat. *Reflective Practice*, **1**, 5–9.

Johns, C. (2004) Becoming a transformational leader through reflection. *Reflections on Nursing Leadership*, **30**(2), 24–26, 38.

Joyce-McCoach, J. and Smith, K. (2016) A teaching model for health professionals learning reflective practice. *Procedia – Social and Behavioural Sciences*, **228**, 265–271.

Karpman, S (1968) Fairy tales and script drama analysis. *Transactional Analysis Journal*, **7**, 26.

Lewin, K. (1946) Force field analysis, in *The 1973 Annual Handbook for Group Facilitators* (eds J.E. Jones and J.W. Pfeiffer). University Associates, San Diego, CA, pp. 111–113.

Lewin, K. (1951) *Field Theory in Social Science*. Harper and Row, New York.

Luft, J. and Ingham, H. (1955) *The Johari Window: A Graphic Model of Awareness in Interpersonal Relations*. University of California Western Training Lab, San Diego.

Oelofsen, N. (2012) Using reflective practice in frontline nursing. *Nursing Times*, **108**(24) 22–24.

Schön, D. (1983) *The Reflective Practitioner: How Professionals Think in Action.*, Basic Books, New York.

Further Reading

Bolton, G. (2005) *Reflective Practice:Writing and Professional Development*, 2nd edn. Sage, London.

Boud, D., Keogh, R. and Walker, D. (1985) *Reflection: Turning Experience into Learning.* Routledge, London.

Bradbury, H., Frost, N., Kilminster, S. and Zukas, M. (2009) *Beyond Reflective Practice: New Approaches to Professional Lifelong Learning.* Routledge, London.

Dewey, J. (1933) *How We Think: A Restatement of the Relation of Reflective Thinking to the Educative Process.* Heath, Boston, MA.

Johns, C. (1995) Framing learning through reflection within Carper's fundamental ways of knowing in nursing. *Journal of Advanced Nursing*, **22**(2), 226–234.

Kolb, D.A. (1984) *Experiential Learning: Experience as the Source of Learning and Development.* Prentice-Hall, New Jersey.

Thomson, S. and Thomson, N. (2008) *The Critically Reflective Practitioner.* Palgrave Macmillan, London.

Reflective models

Allan, H. DEBRIEF: a reflective tool for workplace based learning. Available at: http://educatingtrainers.blogspot.co.uk/search/label/debrief

Atkins, S. and Murphy, K. (1994) Reflective practice. *Nursing Standard*, **8**(39), 49–54.

Barksby, J. (2015) REFLECT: a new model of reflection for clinical practice. *Nursing Times*, **111**(34/35), 21–23.

Driscoll, J. (2006) Reflective practice for practise – a framework of structured reflection for clinical areas. *Senior Nurse*, **14**(1), 47–50.

Gibbs, G. (1988) *Learning by Doing: A guide to teaching and learning methods.* Oxford Brookes University, Oxford.

Johns, C. (2000).*Becoming a Reflective Practitioner.* Blackwell Science, Oxford.

Peters, J. (1991) Strategies for reflective practice. Professional development for educators of Adults, in *New Directions for Adult and Continuing Education*, No. 51 (ed. R. Brockett). Jossey-Bass, San Francisco, pp. 91–95.

Schön, D. (1991) *The Reflective Practitioner.* Ashgate Publishing, Aldershot.

Index

How to Survive Dental Performance Difficulties, First Edition. Janine Brooks.
© 2018 John Wiley & Sons Ltd. Published 2018 by John Wiley & Sons Ltd.